WORLD HEALTH ORGANIZATION

BASIC DOCUMENTS

Forty-fifth Edition

Including amendments adopted
up to 31 December 2004

GENEVA

2005

WHO Library Cataloguing in Publication Data

World Health Organization
    Basic documents – 45th ed.

    Including amendments adopted up to 31 December 2004.

    1.World Health Organization   2.Constitution and bylaws   I.Title.

    ISBN 92 4 165045 1   (NLM Classification: WA 540 MW6)

Printed in Switzerland

For index, see page 181
CONTENTS

(Continued overleaf)

APPENDICES

Note: In accordance with resolution WHA57.8, the use of one gender in
    Basic documents shall be considered as including a reference to the
    other unless the context otherwise requires.

CONSTITUTION
OF THE WORLD HEALTH ORGANIZATION[1]

THE STATES Parties to this Constitution declare, in conformity with the Charter of the United Nations, that the following principles are basic to the happiness, harmonious relations and security of all peoples:

Health is a state of complete physical, mental and social well-being and not merely the absence of disease or infirmity.

The enjoyment of the highest attainable standard of health is one of the fundamental rights of every human being without distinction of race, religion, political belief, economic or social condition.

The health of all peoples is fundamental to the attainment of peace and security and is dependent upon the fullest co-operation of individuals and States.

The achievement of any State in the promotion and protection of health is of value to all.

Unequal development in different countries in the promotion of health and control of disease, especially communicable disease, is a common danger.

Healthy development of the child is of basic importance; the ability to live harmoniously in a changing total environment is essential to such development.

The extension to all peoples of the benefits of medical, psychological and related knowledge is essential to the fullest attainment of health.

Informed opinion and active co-operation on the part of the public are of the utmost importance in the improvement of the health of the people.

Governments have a responsibility for the health of their peoples which can be fulfilled only by the provision of adequate health and social measures.

ACCEPTING THESE PRINCIPLES, and for the purpose of co-operation among themselves and with others to promote and protect the health of all peoples, the Contracting Parties agree to the present Constitution and

---

[1] The Constitution was adopted by the International Health Conference held in New York from 19 June to 22 July 1946, signed on 22 July 1946 by the representatives of 61 States (*Off. Rec. Wld Hlth Org.*, **2**, 100), and entered into force on 7 April 1948. Amendments adopted by the Twenty-sixth, Twenty-ninth and Thirty-ninth World Health Assemblies (resolutions WHA26.37, WHA29.38 and WHA39.6) came into force on 3 February 1977, 20 January 1984 and 11 July 1994 respectively and are incorporated in the present text.

hereby establish the World Health Organization as a specialized agency within the terms of Article 57 of the Charter of the United Nations.

CHAPTER I – OBJECTIVE

Article 1

The objective of the World Health Organization (hereinafter called the Organization) shall be the attainment by all peoples of the highest possible level of health.

CHAPTER II – FUNCTIONS

Article 2

In order to achieve its objective, the functions of the Organization shall be:

(*a*) to act as the directing and co-ordinating authority on international health work;

(*b*) to establish and maintain effective collaboration with the United Nations, specialized agencies, governmental health administrations, professional groups and such other organizations as may be deemed appropriate;

(*c*) to assist Governments, upon request, in strengthening health services;

(*d*) to furnish appropriate technical assistance and, in emergencies, necessary aid upon the request or acceptance of Governments;

(*e*) to provide or assist in providing, upon the request of the United Nations, health services and facilities to special groups, such as the peoples of trust territories;

(*f*) to establish and maintain such administrative and technical services as may be required, including epidemiological and statistical services;

(*g*) to stimulate and advance work to eradicate epidemic, endemic and other diseases;

(*h*) to promote, in co-operation with other specialized agencies where necessary, the prevention of accidental injuries;

(*i*) to promote, in co-operation with other specialized agencies where necessary, the improvement of nutrition, housing, sanitation, recreation, economic or working conditions and other aspects of environmental hygiene;

(*j*) to promote co-operation among scientific and professional groups which contribute to the advancement of health;

(*k*) to propose conventions, agreements and regulations, and make recommendations with respect to international health matters and to perform such duties as may be assigned thereby to the Organization and are consistent with its objective;

(*l*) to promote maternal and child health and welfare and to foster the ability to live harmoniously in a changing total environment;

(*m*) to foster activities in the field of mental health, especially those affecting the harmony of human relations;

(*n*) to promote and conduct research in the field of health;

(*o*) to promote improved standards of teaching and training in the health, medical and related professions;

(*p*) to study and report on, in co-operation with other specialized agencies where necessary, administrative and social techniques affecting public health and medical care from preventive and curative points of view, including hospital services and social security;

(*q*) to provide information, counsel and assistance in the field of health;

(*r*) to assist in developing an informed public opinion among all peoples on matters of health;

(*s*) to establish and revise as necessary international nomenclatures of diseases, of causes of death and of public health practices;

(*t*) to standardize diagnostic procedures as necessary;

(*u*) to develop, establish and promote international standards with respect to food, biological, pharmaceutical and similar products;

(*v*) generally to take all necessary action to attain the objective of the Organization.

CHAPTER III – MEMBERSHIP AND ASSOCIATE MEMBERSHIP

Article 3

Membership in the Organization shall be open to all States.

Article 4

Members of the United Nations may become Members of the Organization by signing or otherwise accepting this Constitution in accordance with the provisions of Chapter XIX and in accordance with their constitutional processes.

Article 5

The States whose Governments have been invited to send observers to the International Health Conference held in New York, 1946, may become

Members by signing or otherwise accepting this Constitution in accordance with the provisions of Chapter XIX and in accordance with their constitutional processes provided that such signature or acceptance shall be completed before the first session of the Health Assembly.

Article 6

Subject to the conditions of any agreement between the United Nations and the Organization, approved pursuant to Chapter XVI, States which do not become Members in accordance with Articles 4 and 5 may apply to become Members and shall be admitted as Members when their application has been approved by a simple majority vote of the Health Assembly.

Article 7[1]

If a Member fails to meet its financial obligations to the Organization or in other exceptional circumstances, the Health Assembly may, on such conditions as it thinks proper, suspend the voting privileges and services to which a Member is entitled. The Health Assembly shall have the authority to restore such voting privileges and services.

Article 8

Territories or groups of territories which are not responsible for the conduct of their international relations may be admitted as Associate Members by the Health Assembly upon application made on behalf of such territory or group of territories by the Member or other authority having responsibility for their international relations. Representatives of Associate Members to the Health Assembly should be qualified by their technical competence in the field of health and should be chosen from the native population. The nature and extent of the rights and obligations of Associate Members shall be determined by the Health Assembly.

CHAPTER IV – ORGANS

Article 9

The work of the Organization shall be carried out by:

(a) The World Health Assembly (herein called the Health Assembly);
(b) The Executive Board (hereinafter called the Board);
(c) The Secretariat.

---

[1] The amendment to this Article adopted by the Eighteenth World Health Assembly (resolution WHA18.48) has not yet come into force.

CHAPTER V – THE WORLD HEALTH ASSEMBLY

Article 10

The Health Assembly shall be composed of delegates representing Members.

Article 11

Each Member shall be represented by not more than three delegates, one of whom shall be designated by the Member as chief delegate. These delegates should be chosen from among persons most qualified by their technical competence in the field of health, preferably representing the national health administration of the Member.

Article 12

Alternates and advisers may accompany delegates.

Article 13

The Health Assembly shall meet in regular annual session and in such special sessions as may be necessary. Special sessions shall be convened at the request of the Board or of a majority of the Members.

Article 14

The Health Assembly, at each annual session, shall select the country or region in which the next annual session shall be held, the Board subsequently fixing the place. The Board shall determine the place where a special session shall be held.

Article 15

The Board, after consultation with the Secretary-General of the United Nations, shall determine the date of each annual and special session.

Article 16

The Health Assembly shall elect its President and other officers at the beginning of each annual session. They shall hold office until their successors are elected.

Article 17

The Health Assembly shall adopt its own rules of procedure.

Article 18

The functions of the Health Assembly shall be:

(*a*) to determine the policies of the Organization;

(*b*) to name the Members entitled to designate a person to serve on the Board;

(*c*) to appoint the Director-General;

(*d*) to review and approve reports and activities of the Board and of the Director-General and to instruct the Board in regard to matters upon which action, study, investigation or report may be considered desirable;

(*e*) to establish such committees as may be considered necessary for the work of the Organization;

(*f*) to supervise the financial policies of the Organization and to review and approve the budget;

(*g*) to instruct the Board and the Director-General to bring to the attention of Members and of international organizations, governmental or non-governmental, any matter with regard to health which the Health Assembly may consider appropriate;

(*h*) to invite any organization, international or national, governmental or non-governmental, which has responsibilities related to those of the Organization, to appoint representatives to participate, without right of vote, in its meetings or in those of the committees and conferences convened under its authority, on conditions prescribed by the Health Assembly; but in the case of national organizations, invitations shall be issued only with the consent of the Government concerned;

(*i*) to consider recommendations bearing on health made by the General Assembly, the Economic and Social Council, the Security Council or Trusteeship Council of the United Nations, and to report to them on the steps taken by the Organization to give effect to such recommendations;

(*j*) to report to the Economic and Social Council in accordance with any agreement between the Organization and the United Nations;

(*k*) to promote and conduct research in the field of health by the personnel of the Organization, by the establishment of its own institutions or by co-operation with official or non-official institutions of any Member with the consent of its Government;

(*l*) to establish such other institutions as it may consider desirable;

(*m*) to take any other appropriate action to further the objective of the Organization.

Article 19

The Health Assembly shall have authority to adopt conventions or agreements with respect to any matter within the competence of the Organization. A two-thirds vote of the Health Assembly shall be required for the adoption of such conventions or agreements, which shall come into force for each Member when accepted by it in accordance with its constitutional processes.

Article 20

Each Member undertakes that it will, within eighteen months after the adoption by the Health Assembly of a convention or agreement, take action relative to the acceptance of such convention or agreement. Each Member shall notify the Director-General of the action taken, and if it does not accept such convention or agreement within the time limit, it will furnish a statement of the reasons for non-acceptance. In case of acceptance, each Member agrees to make an annual report to the Director-General in accordance with Chapter XIV.

Article 21

The Health Assembly shall have authority to adopt regulations concerning:

(*a*) sanitary and quarantine requirements and other procedures designed to prevent the international spread of disease;

(*b*) nomenclatures with respect to diseases, causes of death and public health practices;

(*c*) standards with respect to diagnostic procedures for international use;

(*d*) standards with respect to the safety, purity and potency of biological, pharmaceutical and similar products moving in international commerce;

(*e*) advertising and labelling of biological, pharmaceutical and similar products moving in international commerce.

Article 22

Regulations adopted pursuant to Article 21 shall come into force for all Members after due notice has been given of their adoption by the Health Assembly except for such Members as may notify the Director-General of rejection or reservations within the period stated in the notice.

Article 23

The Health Assembly shall have authority to make recommendations to Members with respect to any matter within the competence of the Organization.

CHAPTER VI – THE EXECUTIVE BOARD

Article 24[1]

The Board shall consist of thirty-two persons designated by as many Members. The Health Assembly, taking into account an equitable geographical distribution, shall elect the Members entitled to designate a person to serve on the Board, provided that, of such Members, not less than three shall be elected from each of the regional organizations established pursuant to Article 44. Each of these Members should appoint to the Board a person technically qualified in the field of health, who may be accompanied by alternates and advisers.

Article 25[1]

These Members shall be elected for three years and may be re-elected, provided that of the Members elected at the first session of the Health Assembly held after the coming into force of the amendment to this Constitution increasing the membership of the Board from thirty-one to thirty-two the term of office of the additional Member elected shall, insofar as may be necessary, be of such lesser duration as shall facilitate the election of at least one Member from each regional organization in each year.

Article 26

The Board shall meet at least twice a year and shall determine the place of each meeting.

Article 27

The Board shall elect its Chairman from among its members and shall adopt its own rules of procedure.

Article 28

The functions of the Board shall be:

(*a*) to give effect to the decisions and policies of the Health Assembly;

(*b*) to act as the executive organ of the Health Assembly;

---

[1] The amendment to this Article by the Fifty-first World Health Assembly (resolution WHA51.23) has not yet come into force.

(c) to perform any other functions entrusted to it by the Health Assembly;

(d) to advise the Health Assembly on questions referred to it by that body and on matters assigned to the Organization by conventions, agreements and regulations;

(e) to submit advice or proposals to the Health Assembly on its own initiative;

(f) to prepare the agenda of meetings of the Health Assembly;

(g) to submit to the Health Assembly for consideration and approval a general programme of work covering a specific period;

(h) to study all questions within its competence;

(i) to take emergency measures within the functions and financial resources of the Organization to deal with events requiring immediate action. In particular it may authorize the Director-General to take the necessary steps to combat epidemics, to participate in the organization of health relief to victims of a calamity and to undertake studies and research the urgency of which has been drawn to the attention of the Board by any Member or by the Director-General.

Article 29

The Board shall exercise on behalf of the whole Health Assembly the powers delegated to it by that body.

CHAPTER VII – THE SECRETARIAT

Article 30

The Secretariat shall comprise the Director-General and such technical and administrative staff as the Organization may require.

Article 31

The Director-General shall be appointed by the Health Assembly on the nomination of the Board on such terms as the Health Assembly may determine. The Director-General, subject to the authority of the Board, shall be the chief technical and administrative officer of the Organization.

Article 32

The Director-General shall be *ex-officio* Secretary of the Health Assembly, of the Board, of all commissions and committees of the Organization and of conferences convened by it. He may delegate these functions.

Article 33

The Director-General or his representative may establish a procedure by agreement with Members, permitting him, for the purpose of discharging his duties, to have direct access to their various departments, especially to their health administrations and to national health organizations, governmental or non-governmental. He may also establish direct relations with international organizations whose activities come within the competence of the Organization. He shall keep regional offices informed on all matters involving their respective areas.

Article 34

The Director-General shall prepare and submit to the Board the financial statements and budget estimates of the Organization.

Article 35

The Director-General shall appoint the staff of the Secretariat in accordance with staff regulations established by the Health Assembly. The paramount consideration in the employment of the staff shall be to assure that the efficiency, integrity and internationally representative character of the Secretariat shall be maintained at the highest level. Due regard shall be paid also to the importance of recruiting the staff on as wide a geographical basis as possible.

Article 36

The conditions of service of the staff of the Organization shall conform as far as possible with those of other United Nations organizations.

Article 37

In the performance of their duties the Director-General and the staff shall not seek or receive instructions from any government or from any authority external to the Organization. They shall refrain from any action which might reflect on their position as international officers. Each Member of the Organization on its part undertakes to respect the exclusively international character of the Director-General and the staff and not to seek to influence them.

CHAPTER VIII – COMMITTEES

Article 38

The Board shall establish such committees as the Health Assembly may direct and, on its own initiative or on the proposal of the Director-General, may establish any other committees considered desirable to serve any purpose within the competence of the Organization.

Article 39

The Board, from time to time and in any event annually, shall review the necessity for continuing each committee.

Article 40

The Board may provide for the creation of or the participation by the Organization in joint or mixed committees with other organizations and for the representation of the Organization in committees established by such other organizations.

CHAPTER IX – CONFERENCES

Article 41

The Health Assembly or the Board may convene local, general, technical or other special conferences to consider any matter within the competence of the Organization and may provide for the representation at such conferences of international organizations and, with the consent of the Government concerned, of national organizations, governmental or non-governmental. The manner of such representation shall be determined by the Health Assembly or the Board.

Article 42

The Board may provide for representation of the Organization at conferences in which the Board considers that the Organization has an interest.

CHAPTER X – HEADQUARTERS

Article 43

The location of the headquarters of the Organization shall be determined by the Health Assembly after consultation with the United Nations.

CHAPTER XI – REGIONAL ARRANGEMENTS

Article 44

(a) The Health Assembly shall from time to time define the geographical areas in which it is desirable to establish a regional organization.

(b) The Health Assembly may, with the consent of a majority of the Members situated within each area so defined, establish a regional organization to meet the special needs of such area. There shall not be more than one regional organization in each area.

Article 45

Each regional organization shall be an integral part of the Organization in accordance with this Constitution.

Article 46

Each regional organization shall consist of a regional committee and a regional office.

Article 47

Regional committees shall be composed of representatives of the Member States and Associate Members in the region concerned. Territories or groups of territories within the region, which are not responsible for the conduct of their international relations and which are not Associate Members, shall have the right to be represented and to participate in regional committees. The nature and extent of the rights and obligations of these territories or groups of territories in regional committees shall be determined by the Health Assembly in consultation with the Member or other authority having responsibility for the international relations of these territories and with the Member States in the region.

Article 48

Regional committees shall meet as often as necessary and shall determine the place of each meeting.

Article 49

Regional committees shall adopt their own rules of procedure.

Article 50

The functions of the regional committee shall be:

(*a*) to formulate policies governing matters of an exclusively regional character;

(*b*) to supervise the activities of the regional office;

(*c*) to suggest to the regional office the calling of technical conferences and such additional work or investigation in health matters as in the opinion of the regional committee would promote the objective of the Organization within the region;

(*d*) to co-operate with the respective regional committees of the United Nations and with those of other specialized agencies and with other regional international organizations having interests in common with the Organization;

(e) to tender advice, through the Director-General, to the Organization on international health matters which have wider than regional significance;

(f) to recommend additional regional appropriations by the Governments of the respective regions if the proportion of the central budget of the Organization allotted to that region is insufficient for the carrying-out of the regional functions;

(g) such other functions as may be delegated to the regional committee by the Health Assembly, the Board or the Director-General.

Article 51

Subject to the general authority of the Director-General of the Organization, the regional office shall be the administrative organ of the regional committee. It shall, in addition, carry out within the region the decisions of the Health Assembly and of the Board.

Article 52

The head of the regional office shall be the Regional Director appointed by the Board in agreement with the regional committee.

Article 53

The staff of the regional office shall be appointed in a manner to be determined by agreement between the Director-General and the Regional Director.

Article 54

The Pan American Sanitary Organization[1] represented by the Pan American Sanitary Bureau and the Pan American Sanitary Conferences, and all other inter-governmental regional health organizations in existence prior to the date of signature of this Constitution, shall in due course be integrated with the Organization. This integration shall be effected as soon as practicable through common action based on mutual consent of the competent authorities expressed through the organizations concerned.

CHAPTER XII – BUDGET AND EXPENSES

Article 55

The Director-General shall prepare and submit to the Board the budget estimates of the Organization. The Board shall consider and submit to the Health Assembly such budget estimates, together with any recommendations the Board may deem advisable.

---

[1] Renamed "Pan American Health Organization" by decision of the XV Pan American Sanitary Conference, September-October 1958.

Article 56

Subject to any agreement between the Organization and the United Nations, the Health Assembly shall review and approve the budget estimates and shall apportion the expenses among the Members in accordance with a scale to be fixed by the Health Assembly.

Article 57

The Health Assembly or the Board acting on behalf of the Health Assembly may accept and administer gifts and bequests made to the Organization provided that the conditions attached to such gifts or bequests are acceptable to the Health Assembly or the Board and are consistent with the objective and policies of the Organization.

Article 58

A special fund to be used at the discretion of the Board shall be established to meet emergencies and unforeseen contingencies.

CHAPTER XIII – VOTING

Article 59

Each Member shall have one vote in the Health Assembly.

Article 60

(*a*) Decisions of the Health Assembly on important questions shall be made by a two-thirds majority of the Members present and voting. These questions shall include: the adoption of conventions or agreements; the approval of agreements bringing the Organization into relation with the United Nations and inter-governmental organizations and agencies in accordance with Articles 69, 70 and 72; amendments to this Constitution.

(*b*) Decisions on other questions, including the determination of additional categories of questions to be decided by a two-thirds majority, shall be made by a majority of the Members present and voting.

(*c*) Voting on analogous matters in the Board and in committees of the Organization shall be made in accordance with paragraphs (*a*) and (*b*) of this Article.

CHAPTER XIV – REPORTS SUBMITTED BY STATES

Article 61

Each Member shall report annually to the Organization on the action taken and progress achieved in improving the health of its people.

Article 62

Each Member shall report annually on the action taken with respect to recommendations made to it by the Organization and with respect to conventions, agreements and regulations.

Article 63

Each Member shall communicate promptly to the Organization important laws, regulations, official reports and statistics pertaining to health which have been published in the State concerned.

Article 64

Each Member shall provide statistical and epidemiological reports in a manner to be determined by the Health Assembly.

Article 65

Each Member shall transmit upon the request of the Board such additional information pertaining to health as may be practicable.

CHAPTER XV – LEGAL CAPACITY, PRIVILEGES AND IMMUNITIES

Article 66

The Organization shall enjoy in the territory of each Member such legal capacity as may be necessary for the fulfilment of its objective and for the exercise of its functions.

Article 67

(*a*) The Organization shall enjoy in the territory of each Member such privileges and immunities as may be necessary for the fulfilment of its objective and for the exercise of its functions.

(*b*) Representatives of Members, persons designated to serve on the Board and technical and administrative personnel of the Organization shall similarly enjoy such privileges and immunities as are necessary for the independent exercise of their functions in connexion with the Organization.

Article 68

Such legal capacity, privileges and immunities shall be defined in a separate agreement to be prepared by the Organization in consultation with the Secretary-General of the United Nations and concluded between the Members.

CHAPTER XVI – RELATIONS WITH OTHER ORGANIZATIONS

Article 69

The Organization shall be brought into relation with the United Nations as one of the specialized agencies referred to in Article 57 of the Charter of the United Nations. The agreement or agreements bringing the Organization into relation with the United Nations shall be subject to approval by a two-thirds vote of the Health Assembly.

Article 70

The Organization shall establish effective relations and co-operate closely with such other inter-governmental organizations as may be desirable. Any formal agreement entered into with such organizations shall be subject to approval by a two-thirds vote of the Health Assembly.

Article 71

The Organization may, on matters within its competence, make suitable arrangements for consultation and co-operation with non-governmental international organizations and, with the consent of the Government concerned, with national organizations, governmental or non-governmental.

Article 72

Subject to the approval by a two-thirds vote of the Health Assembly, the Organization may take over from any other international organization or agency whose purpose and activities lie within the field of competence of the Organization such functions, resources and obligations as may be conferred upon the Organization by international agreement or by mutually acceptable arrangements entered into between the competent authorities of the respective organizations.

CHAPTER XVII – AMENDMENTS

Article 73

Texts of proposed amendments to this Constitution shall be communicated by the Director-General to Members at least six months in advance of their consideration by the Health Assembly. Amendments shall come into force for all Members when adopted by a two-thirds vote of the Health Assembly and accepted by two-thirds of the Members in accordance with their respective constitutional processes.

CHAPTER XVIII – INTERPRETATION

Article 74 [1]

The Chinese, English, French, Russian and Spanish texts of this Constitution shall be regarded as equally authentic.

Article 75

Any question or dispute concerning the interpretation or application of this Constitution which is not settled by negotiation or by the Health Assembly shall be referred to the International Court of Justice in conformity with the Statute of the Court, unless the parties concerned agree on another mode of settlement.

Article 76

Upon authorization by the General Assembly of the United Nations or upon authorization in accordance with any agreement between the Organization and the United Nations, the Organization may request the International Court of Justice for an advisory opinion on any legal question arising within the competence of the Organization.

Article 77

The Director-General may appear before the Court on behalf of the Organization in connexion with any proceedings arising out of any such request for an advisory opinion. He shall make arrangements for the presentation of the case before the Court, including arrangements for the argument of different views on the question.

CHAPTER XIX – ENTRY-INTO-FORCE

Article 78

Subject to the provisions of Chapter III, this Constitution shall remain open to all States for signature or acceptance.

Article 79

(a) States may become parties to this Constitution by:

(i)   signature without reservation as to approval;

(ii) signature subject to approval followed by acceptance; or

(iii) acceptance.

---

[1] The amendment to this Article adopted by the Thirty-first World Health Assembly (resolution WHA31.18) has not yet come into force.

(*b*) Acceptance shall be effected by the deposit of a formal instrument with the Secretary-General of the United Nations.

Article 80

This Constitution shall come into force when twenty-six Members of the United Nations have become parties to it in accordance with the provisions of Article 79.

Article 81

In accordance with Article 102 of the Charter of the United Nations, the Secretary-General of the United Nations will register this Constitution when it has been signed without reservation as to approval on behalf of one State or upon deposit of the first instrument of acceptance.

Article 82

The Secretary-General of the United Nations will inform States parties to this Constitution of the date when it has come into force. He will also inform them of the dates when other States have become parties to this Constitution.

IN FAITH WHEREOF the undersigned representatives, having been duly authorized for that purpose, sign this Constitution.

DONE in the City of New York this twenty-second day of July 1946, in a single copy in the Chinese, English, French, Russian and Spanish languages, each text being equally authentic. The original texts shall be deposited in the archives of the United Nations. The Secretary-General of the United Nations will send certified copies to each of the Governments represented at the Conference.

RIGHTS AND OBLIGATIONS OF ASSOCIATE MEMBERS AND OTHER TERRITORIES

1. Health Assembly and Executive Board[1]

Whereas Article 8 of the Constitution of the World Health Organization provides that the nature and extent of the rights and obligations of Associate Members shall be determined by the Health Assembly, and

Whereas there is need for further study in connexion with Articles 8 and 47 of the Constitution of the rights and obligations in regional organizations of Associate Members and of territories or groups of territories which are not responsible for the conduct of their international relations and which are not Associate Members,

The First World Health Assembly

RESOLVES

1. that Associate Members shall have the right:

(i) to participate without vote in the deliberations of the Health Assembly and its main committees;

(i) to participate with vote and to hold office in other committees or subcommittees of the Assembly, except the General Committee, the Committee on Credentials, and the Nominations Committee;

(iii) to participate equally with Members, subject to the limitation on voting in paragraph (i) above, in matters pertaining to the conduct of business of meetings of the Assembly and its committees, in accordance with Rules 50 to 70, and 85 to 86, of the Rules of Procedure of the Assembly;

(iv) to propose items for inclusion in the provisional agenda of the Assembly;

(v) to receive equally with Members all notices, documents, reports and records;

(vi) to participate equally with Members in the procedure for convening special sessions;

---

[1] Text adopted by the First World Health Assembly on 21 July 1948 (*Off. Rec. Wld Hlth Org.*, **13**, 100, 337). (The numbers of the Rules of Procedure mentioned in paragraph 1 (iii) have been changed to agree with the revised version of the Rules as reproduced on p. 122.)

2. that Associate Members shall have the right, equally with Members, to submit proposals to the Executive Board, and to participate, in accordance with regulations established by the Board, in committees established by it, but they shall not be eligible for membership on the Board;

3. that Associate Members shall be subject to the same obligations as Members, except that the difference in their status shall be taken into account in determining the amount of their contribution to the budget of the Organization;

4. that the Executive Board be requested to submit a report with recommendations to the next Health Assembly, taking into account Article 47 of the Constitution and any comments or recommendations from Members and from regional organizations concerning the rights and obligations in regional organizations of Associate Members and of territories or groups of territories which are not responsible for the conduct of their international relations and which are not Associate Members, the report to be transmitted to the Members at least two months in advance of the convening of the Assembly.

2. Regional Organizations[1]

The Second World Health Assembly,

Having regard to Articles 8 and 47 of the Constitution; and

Having regard to paragraph 4 of the resolution of the First World Health Assembly concerning the rights and obligations of Associate Members;[2] and

Having regard to the reports of the Executive Board at its second and third sessions;[3] and

Having regard to a statement[4] concerning the Pan American Sanitary Organization,[5]

RESOLVES AS FOLLOWS:

1. For the purposes of Article 47 of the Constitution, States Members in a region shall be deemed to be those States Members having their seat of government within the region;

---

[1] Text adopted by the Second World Health Assembly on 30 June 1949 (resolution WHA2.103). The rights and obligations of Associate Members were further considered by the Fifth, Sixth, Seventh, Ninth and Tenth World Health Assemblies, and by the Executive Board at its ninth, tenth, eleventh, thirteenth, fifteenth and nineteenth sessions but have remained unchanged. The relevant resolutions will be found in the *Handbook of Resolutions and Decisions of the World Health Assembly and the Executive Board,* Volume I, section 6.2.2. As regards participation in the Regional Committee for Africa of Members not having their seat of government within the Region, see resolution WHA28.37.
[2] See above.
[3] *Off. Rec. Wld Hlth Org.,* **14**, 26, 54; **17**, 17.
[4] *Off. Rec. Wld Hlth Org.,* **21**, 384.
[5] Renamed "Pan American Health Organization" by decision of the XV Pan American Sanitary Conference, September-October 1958.

2. Those States Members not having their seat of government within the region, which (a) either by reason of their Constitution consider certain territories or groups of territories in the region as part of their national territory, or (b) are responsible for the conduct of the international relations of territories or groups of territories within the region, shall participate as Members of the regional committee, in which case they shall have all the rights, privileges and obligations of Member States in the region, but with only one vote for all the territories or groups of territories in the region, as defined in (a) and (b) above;

3. (1) Territories or groups of territories in the region which are not responsible for the conduct of their international relations, whether Associate Members or otherwise, may participate in regional committees, in accordance with Articles 8 and 47 of the Constitution;

(2) Associate Members shall have all rights and obligations in the regional organizations, with the exception that they will have no vote in plenary meetings of the regional committee, nor in subdivisions dealing with finance or constitutional matters;

(3) Representatives of Associate Members should be qualified by their technical competence in the field of health and should be chosen from the native population in accordance with Article 8 of the Constitution;

(4) In the case of territories not responsible for the conduct of their international relations and not Associate Members, the rights and obligations in (2) above shall apply subject to consultation between the States Members in a region – as defined in paragraph 1 above – and the Members or other authority having responsibility for the international relations of these territories;

(5) In recommending any additional appropriation under Article 50(*f*) of the Constitution, the regional committee shall take account of the difference in status between States Members, on the one hand, and Associate Members and other territories or groups of territories not responsible for the conduct of their international relations, on the other;

4. In view of the statement made by the Director of the Pan American Sanitary Organization [1] and of the fact that integration between PASO and WHO is still in process, the application of the above recommendation in the American Region shall await the completion of these negotiations for such integration;

---

[1] *Off. Rec. Wld Hlth Org.*, **21**, 384.

5. The Executive Board should keep under review the implementation of these decisions and submit to the Fifth World Health Assembly,[1] at the latest, a report thereon in order that that Assembly might determine what, if any, modifications might be required in the above decisions in the light of experience.

---

[1] See footnote 1 on p. 20.

CONVENTION ON THE PRIVILEGES
AND IMMUNITIES OF THE SPECIALIZED AGENCIES[1]

WHEREAS the General Assembly of the United Nations adopted on 13 February 1946 a resolution contemplating the unification as far as possible of the privileges and immunities enjoyed by the United Nations and by the various specialized agencies; and

WHEREAS consultations concerning the implementation of the aforesaid resolution have taken place between the United Nations and the specialized agencies;

CONSEQUENTLY, by resolution 179 (II) adopted on 21 November 1947, the General Assembly has approved the following Convention, which is submitted to the specialized agencies for acceptance and to every Member of the United Nations and to every other State member of one or more of the specialized agencies for accession.

Article I – Definitions and Scope

Section 1

In this Convention:

(i) The words "standard clauses" refer to the provisions of Articles II to IX.

(ii) The words "specialized agencies" mean:

- (*a*) The International Labour Organisation;
- (*b*) The Food and Agriculture Organization of the United Nations;
- (*c*) The United Nations Educational, Scientific and Cultural Organization;
- (*d*) The International Civil Aviation Organization;
- (*e*) The International Monetary Fund;
- (*f*) The International Bank for Reconstruction and Development;
- (*g*) The World Health Organization;
- (*h*) The Universal Postal Union;
- (*i*) The International Telecommunication Union; and

---

[1] Adopted by the First World Health Assembly on 17 July 1948 (*Off. Rec. Wld Hlth Org.*, **13**, 97, 332).

(*j*) Any other agency in relationship with the United Nations in accordance with Articles 57 and 63 of the Charter.

(iii) The word "Convention" means, in relation to any particular specialized agency, the standard clauses as modified by the final (or revised) text of the annex transmitted by that agency in accordance with sections 36 and 38.

(iv) For the purposes of article III, the words "property and assets" shall also include property and funds administered by a specialized agency in furtherance of its constitutional functions.

(v) For the purposes of articles V and VII, the expression "representatives of members" shall be deemed to include all representatives, alternates, advisers, technical experts and secretaries of delegations.

(vi) In sections 13, 14, 15 and 25, the expression "meetings convened by a specialized agency" means meetings: (1) of its assembly and of its executive body (however designated), and (2) of any commission provided for in its constitution; (3) of any international conference convened by it; and (4) of any committee of any of these bodies.

(vii) The term "executive head" means the principal executive official of the specialized agency in question, whether designated "Director-General" or otherwise.

Section 2

Each State party to this Convention in respect of any specialized agency to which this Convention has become applicable in accordance with section 37 shall accord to, or in connexion with, that agency the privileges and immunities set forth in the standard clauses on the conditions specified therein, subject to any modification of those clauses contained in the provisions of the final (or revised) annex relating to that agency and transmitted in accordance with sections 36 or 38.

Article II – Juridical Personality

Section 3

The specialized agencies shall possess juridical personality. They shall have the capacity (a) to contract, (b) to acquire and dispose of immovable and movable property, (c) to institute legal proceedings.

Article III – Property, Funds and Assets

Section 4

The specialized agencies, their property and assets, wherever located and by whomsoever held, shall enjoy immunity from every form of legal process except in so far as in any particular case they have expressly waived their immunity. It is, however, understood that no waiver of immunity shall extend to any measure of execution.

Section 5

The premises of the specialized agencies shall be inviolable. The property and assets of the specialized agencies, wherever located and by whomsoever held, shall be immune from search, requisition, confiscation, expropriation and any other form of interference, whether by executive, administrative, judicial or legislative action.

Section 6

The archives of the specialized agencies, and in general all documents belonging to them or held by them, shall be inviolable, wherever located.

Section 7

Without being restricted by financial controls, regulations or moratoria of any kind:

(*a*) The specialized agencies may hold funds, gold or currency of any kind and operate accounts in any currency;

(*b*) The specialized agencies may freely transfer their funds, gold or currency from one country to another or within any country and convert any currency held by them into any other currency.

Section 8

Each specialized agency shall, in exercising its rights under section 7 above, pay due regard to any representations made by the Government of any State party to this Convention in so far as it is considered that effect can be given to such representations without detriment to the interests of the agency.

Section 9

The specialized agencies, their assets, income and other property shall be:

(*a*) Exempt from all direct taxes; it is understood, however, that the specialized agencies will not claim exemption from taxes which are, in fact, no more than charges for public utility services;

(*b*) Exempt from customs duties and prohibitions and restrictions on imports and exports in respect of articles imported or exported by the specialized agencies for their official use; it is understood, however, that articles imported under such exemption will not be sold in the country into which they were imported except under conditions agreed to with the Government of that country;

(*c*) Exempt from duties and prohibitions and restrictions on imports and exports in respect of their publications.

Section 10

While the specialized agencies will not, as a general rule, claim exemption from excise duties and from taxes on the sale of movable and immovable property which form part of the price to be paid, nevertheless when the specialized agencies are making important purchases for official use of property on which such duties and taxes have been charged or are chargeable, States parties to this Convention will, whenever possible, make appropriate administrative arrangements for the remission or return of the amount of duty or tax.

Article IV – Facilities in respect of Communications

Section 11

Each specialized agency shall enjoy, in the territory of each State party to this Convention in respect of that agency, for its official communications, treatment not less favourable than that accorded by the Government of such State to any other Government, including the latter's diplomatic mission, in the matter of priorities, rates and taxes on mails, cables, telegrams, radiograms, telephotos, telephone and other communications, and press rates for information to the press and radio.

Section 12

No censorship shall be applied to the official correspondence and other official communications of the specialized agencies.

The specialized agencies shall have the right to use codes and to dispatch and receive correspondence by courier or in sealed bags, which shall have the same immunities and privileges as diplomatic couriers and bags.

Nothing in this section shall be construed to preclude the adoption of appropriate security precautions to be determined by agreement between a State party to this Convention and a specialized agency.

Article V – Representatives of Members

Section 13

Representatives of members at meetings convened by a specialized agency shall, while exercising their functions and during their journeys to and from the place of meeting, enjoy the following privileges and immunities:

(*a*) Immunity from personal arrest or detention and from seizure of their personal baggage, and in respect of words spoken or written and all acts done by them in their official capacity, immunity from legal process of every kind;

(*b*) Inviolability for all papers and documents;

(*c*) The right to use codes and to receive papers or correspondence by courier or in sealed bags;

(*d*) Exemption in respect of themselves and their spouses from immigration restrictions, aliens' registration or national service obligations in the State which they are visiting or through which they are passing in the exercise of their functions;

(*e*) The same facilities in respect of currency or exchange restrictions as are accorded to representatives of foreign Governments on temporary official missions;

(*f*) The same immunities and facilities in respect of their personal baggage as are accorded to members of comparable rank of diplomatic missions.

Section 14

In order to secure for the representatives of members of the specialized agencies at meetings convened by them complete freedom of speech and complete independence in the discharge of their duties, the immunity from legal process in respect of words spoken or written and all acts done by them in discharging their duties shall continue to be accorded, notwithstanding that the persons concerned are no longer engaged in the discharge of such duties.

Section 15

Where the incidence of any form of taxation depends upon residence, periods during which the representatives of members of the specialized agencies at meetings convened by them are present in a Member State for the discharge of their duties shall not be considered as periods of residence.

Section 16

Privileges and immunities are accorded to the representatives of members, not for the personal benefit of the individuals themselves, but in order to safeguard the independent exercise of their functions in connexion with the specialized agencies. Consequently, a member not only has the right but is under a duty to waive the immunity of its representatives in any case where, in the opinion of the member, the immunity would impede the course of justice, and where it can be waived without prejudice to the purpose for which the immunity is accorded.

Section 17

The provisions of sections 13,14 and 15 are not applicable in relation to the authorities of a State of which the person is a national or of which he is or has been a representative.

Article VI – Officials

Section 18[1]

Each specialized agency will specify the categories of officials to which the provisions of this article and of article VIII shall apply. It shall communicate them to the Governments of all States parties to this Convention in respect of that agency and to the Secretary-General of the United Nations. The names of the officials included in these categories shall from time to time be made known to the above-mentioned Governments.

Section 19

Officials of the specialized agencies shall:

(a) Be immune from legal process in respect of words spoken or written and all acts performed by them in their official capacity;

---

[1] The following resolution (WHA12.41) was adopted by the Twelfth World Health Assembly on 28 May 1959:

The Twelfth World Health Assembly,

Considering Section 18 of Article VI of the Convention on the Privileges and Immunities of the Specialized Agencies which requires that each specialized agency will specify the categories of officials to which the provisions of that Article and Article VIII shall apply; and

Considering the practice hitherto followed by the World Health Organization and under which, in implementing the terms of Section 18 of the Convention, due account has been taken of the provisions of resolution 76 (I) of the General Assembly of the United Nations.

1. CONFIRMS this practice; and

2. APPROVES the granting of the privileges and immunities referred to in Articles VI and VIII of the Convention on the Privileges and Immunities of the Specialized Agencies to all officials of the World Health Organization, with the exception of those who are recruited locally and are assigned to hourly rates.

(*b*) Enjoy the same exemptions from taxation in respect of the salaries and emoluments paid to them by the specialized agencies and on the same conditions as are enjoyed by officials of the United Nations;

(*c*) Be immune, together with their spouses and relatives dependent on them, from immigration restrictions and alien registration;

(*d*) Be accorded the same privileges in respect of exchange facilities as are accorded to officials of comparable rank of diplomatic missions;

(*e*) Be given, together with their spouses and relatives dependent on them, the same repatriation facilities in time of international crises as officials of comparable rank of diplomatic missions;

(*f*) Have the right to import free of duty their furniture and effects at the time of first taking up their post in the country in question.

Section 20

The officials of the specialized agencies shall be exempt from national service obligations, provided that, in relation to the States of which they are nationals, such exemption shall be confined to officials of the specialized agencies whose names have, by reason of their duties, been placed upon a list compiled by the executive head of the specialized agency and approved by the State concerned.

Should other officials of specialized agencies be called up for national service, the State concerned shall, at the request of the specialized agency concerned, grant such temporary deferments in the call-up of such officials as may be necessary to avoid interruption in the continuation of essential work.

Section 21

In addition to the immunities and privileges specified in sections 19 and 20, the executive head of each specialized agency, including any official acting on his behalf during his absence from duty, shall be accorded in respect of himself, his spouse and minor children, the privileges and immunities, exemptions and facilities accorded to diplomatic envoys, in accordance with international law.

Section 22

Privileges and immunities are granted to officials in the interests of the specialized agencies only and not for the personal benefit of the individuals themselves. Each specialized agency shall have the right and the duty to waive the immunity of any official in any case where, in its opinion, the immunity would impede the course of justice and can be waived without prejudice to the interests of the specialized agency.

Section 23

Each specialized agency shall co-operate at all times with the appropriate authorities of Member States to facilitate the proper administration of justice, secure the observance of police regulations and prevent the occurrence of any abuses in connexion with the privileges, immunities and facilities mentioned in this article.

Article VII – Abuses of Privilege

Section 24

If any State party to this Convention considers that there has been an abuse of a privilege or immunity conferred by this Convention, consultations shall be held between that State and the specialized agency concerned to determine whether any such abuse has occurred and, if so, to attempt to ensure that no repetition occurs. If such consultations fail to achieve a result satisfactory to the State and the specialized agency concerned, the question whether an abuse of a privilege or immunity has occurred shall be submitted to the International Court of Justice in accordance with section 32. If the International Court of Justice finds that such an abuse has occurred, the State party to this Convention affected by such abuse shall have the right, after notification to the specialized agency in question, to withhold from the specialized agency concerned the benefits of the privilege or immunity so abused.

Section 25

1. Representatives of members at meetings convened by specialized agencies, while exercising their functions and during their journeys to and from the place of meeting, and officials within the meaning of section 18, shall not be required by the territorial authorities to leave the country in which they are performing their functions on account of any activities by them in their official capacity. In the case, however, of abuse of privileges of residence committed by any such person in activities in that country outside his official functions, he may be required to leave by the Government of that country provided that:

2. (I) Representatives of members, or persons who are entitled to diplomatic immunity under section 21, shall not be required to leave the country

otherwise than in accordance with the diplomatic procedure applicable to diplomatic envoys accredited to that country.

(II) In the case of an official to whom section 21 is not applicable, no order to leave the country shall be issued other than with the approval of the Foreign Minister of the country in question, and such approval shall be given only after consultation with the executive head of the specialized agency concerned; and, if expulsion proceedings are taken against an official, the executive head of the specialized agency shall have the right to appear in such proceedings on behalf of the person against whom they are instituted.

Article VIII – Laissez-passer

Section 26

Officials of the specialized agencies shall be entitled to use the United Nations *laissez-passer* in conformity with administrative arrangements to be concluded between the Secretary-General of the United Nations and the competent authorities of the specialized agencies, to which agencies special powers to issue *laissez-passer* may be delegated. The Secretary-General of the United Nations shall notify each State party to this Convention of each administrative arrangement so concluded.

Section 27

States parties to this Convention shall recognize and accept the United Nations *laissez-passer* issued to officials of the specialized agencies as valid travel documents.

Section 28

Applications for visas, where required, from officials of specialized agencies holding United Nations *laissez-passer*, when accompanied by a certificate that they are travelling on the business of a specialized agency, shall be dealt with as speedily as possible. In addition, such persons shall be granted facilities for speedy travel.

Section 29

Similar facilities to those specified in section 28 shall be accorded to experts and other persons who, though not the holders of United Nations *laissez-passer*, have a certificate that they are travelling on the business of a specialized agency.

Section 30

The executive heads, assistant executive heads, heads of departments and other officials of a rank not lower than head of department of the specialized agencies, travelling on United Nations *laissez-passer* on the business of the specialized agencies, shall be granted the same facilities for travel as are accorded to officials of comparable rank in diplomatic missions.

Article IX – Settlement of Disputes

Section 31

Each specialized agency shall make provision for appropriate modes of settlement of:

(*a*) Disputes arising out of contracts or other disputes of private character to which the specialized agency is a party;

(*b*) Disputes involving any official of a specialized agency who by reason of his official position enjoys immunity, if immunity has not been waived in accordance with the provisions of section 22.

Section 32

All differences arising out of the interpretation or application of the present Convention shall be referred to the International Court of Justice unless in any case it is agreed by the parties to have recourse to another mode of settlement. If a difference arises between one of the specialized agencies on the one hand, and a member on the other hand, a request shall be made for an advisory opinion on any legal question involved in accordance with Article 96 of the Charter and Article 65 of the Statute of the Court and the relevant provisions of the agreements concluded between the United Nations and the specialized agency concerned. The opinion given by the Court shall be accepted as decisive by the parties.

Article X – Annexes and Application to Individual
Specialized Agencies

Section 33

In their application to each specialized agency, the standard clauses shall operate subject to any modifications set forth in the final (or revised) text of the annex relating to that agency, as provided in sections 36 and 38.

Section 34

The provisions of the Convention in relation to any specialized agency must be interpreted in the light of the functions with which that agency is entrusted by its constitutional instrument.

Section 35

Draft annexes I to IX are recommended to the specialized agencies named therein. In the case of any specialized agency not mentioned by name in section 1, the Secretary-General of the United Nations shall transmit to the agency a draft annex recommended by the Economic and Social Council.

Section 36

The final text of each annex shall be that approved by the specialized agency in question in accordance with its constitutional procedure. A copy of the annex as approved by each specialized agency shall be transmitted by the agency in question to the Secretary-General of the United Nations and shall thereupon replace the draft referred to in section 35.

Section 37

The present Convention becomes applicable to each specialized agency when it has transmitted to the Secretary-General of the United Nations the final text of the relevant annex and has informed him that it accepts the standard clauses, as modified by this annex, and undertakes to give effect to sections 8, 18, 22, 23, 24, 31, 32, 42 and 45 (subject to any modification of section 32 which may be found necessary in order to make the final text of the annex consonant with the constitutional instrument of the agency) and any provisions of the annex placing obligations on the agency. The Secretary-General shall communicate to all Members of the United Nations and to other States members of the specialized agencies certified copies of all annexes transmitted to him under this section and of revised annexes transmitted under section 38.

Section 38

If, after the transmission of a final annex under section 36, any specialized agency approves any amendments thereto in accordance with its constitutional procedure, a revised annex shall be transmitted by it to the Secretary-General of the United Nations.

Section 39

The provisions of this Convention shall in no way limit or prejudice the privileges and immunities which have been, or may hereafter be, accorded by any State to any specialized agency by reason of the location in the territory of that State of its headquarters or regional offices. This Convention shall not be deemed to prevent the conclusion between any State party thereto and any specialized agency of supplemental agreements adjusting the provisions of this Convention or extending or curtailing the privileges and immunities thereby granted.

Section 40

It is understood that the standard clauses, as modified by the final text of an annex sent by a specialized agency to the Secretary-General of the United Nations under section 36 (or any revised annex sent under section 38), will be consistent with the provisions of the constitutional instrument then in force of the agency in question, and that if any amendment to that instrument is necessary for the purpose of making the constitutional instrument so consistent, such amendment will have been brought into force in accordance with the constitutional procedure of that agency before the final (or revised) annex is transmitted.

The Convention shall not itself operate so as to abrogate, or derogate from, any provisions of the constitutional instrument of any specialized agency or any rights or obligations which the agency may otherwise have, acquire, or assume.

Article XI – Final Provisions

Section 41

Accession to this Convention by a Member of the United Nations and (subject to section 42) by any State member of a specialized agency shall be effected by deposit with the Secretary-General of the United Nations of an instrument of accession which shall take effect on the date of its deposit.

Section 42

Each specialized agency concerned shall communicate the text of this Convention together with the relevant annexes to those of its members which are not Members of the United Nations and shall invite them to accede thereto in respect of that agency by depositing an instrument of accession to this Convention in respect thereof either with the Secretary-General of the United Nations or with the executive head of the specialized agency.

Section 43

Each State party to this Convention shall indicate in its instrument of accession the specialized agency or agencies in respect of which it undertakes to apply the provisions of this Convention. Each State party to this Convention may by a subsequent written notification to the Secretary-General of the United Nations undertake to apply the provisions of this Convention to one or more further specialized agencies. This notification shall take effect on the date of its receipt by the Secretary-General.

Section 44

This Convention shall enter into force for each State party to this Convention in respect of a specialized agency when it has become applicable to that agency in accordance with section 37 and the State party has undertaken to apply the provisions of the Convention to that agency in accordance with section 43.

Section 45

The Secretary-General of the United Nations shall inform all Members of the United Nations, as well as all members of the specialized agencies, and executive heads of the specialized agencies, of the deposit of each instrument of accession received under section 41 and of subsequent notifications received under section 43. The executive head of a specialized agency shall inform the Secretary-General of the United Nations and the members of the agency concerned of the deposit of any instrument of accession deposited with him under section 42.

Section 46

It is understood that, when an instrument of accession or a subsequent notification is deposited on behalf of any State, this State will be in a position under its own law to give effect to the terms of this Convention, as modified by the final texts of any annexes relating to the agencies covered by such accessions or notifications.

Section 47

1. Subject to the provisions of paragraphs 2 and 3 of this section, each State party to this Convention undertakes to apply this Convention in respect of each specialized agency covered by its accession or subsequent notification, until such time as a revised convention or annex shall have become applicable to that agency and the said State shall have accepted the revised convention or annex. In the case of a revised annex, the acceptance of States shall be by a notification addressed to the Secretary-General of the United Nations, which shall take effect on the date of its receipt by the Secretary-General.

2. Each State party to this Convention, however, which is not, or has ceased to be, a member of a specialized agency, may address a written notification to the Secretary-General of the United Nations and the executive head of the agency concerned to the effect that it intends to withhold from that agency the benefits of this Convention as from a specified date, which shall not be earlier than three months from the date of receipt of the notification.

3. Each State party to this Convention may withhold the benefit of this Convention to any specialized agency which ceases to be in relationship with the United Nations.

4. The Secretary-General of the United Nations shall inform all Member States parties to this Convention of any notification transmitted to him under the provisions of this section.

Section 48

At the request of one-third of the States parties to this Convention, the Secretary-General of the United Nations will convene a conference with a view to its revision.

Section 49

The Secretary-General of the United Nations shall transmit copies of this Convention to each specialized agency and to the Government of each Member of the United Nations.

ANNEX VII - THE WORLD HEALTH ORGANIZATION[1]

In their application to the World Health Organization (hereinafter called "the Organization") the standard clauses shall operate subject to the following modifications:

1. Article V and Section 25, paragraphs 1 and 2 (I), of Article VII shall extend to persons designated to serve on the Executive Board of the Organization, their alternates and advisers, except that any waiver of the immunity of any such persons under Section 16 shall be by the Board.

2. (i) Experts (other than officials coming within the scope of Article VI) serving on committees of, or performing missions for, the Organization shall be accorded the following privileges and immunities so far as is necessary for the effective exercise of their functions, including the time spent on journeys in connexion with service on such committees or missions:

(a) Immunity from personal arrest or seizure of their personal baggage;

(b) In respect of words spoken or written or acts done by them in the performance of their official functions, immunity of legal process of every kind, such immunity to continue notwithstanding that the persons concerned are no longer serving on committees of, or employed on missions for, the Organization;

(c) The same facilities in respect of currency and exchange restrictions and in respect of their personal baggage as are accorded to officials of foreign governments on temporary official missions;

(d) Inviolability for all papers and documents;

(e) For the purpose of their communications with the Organization, the right to use codes and to receive papers or correspondence by courier or in sealed bags.

(ii) The privileges and immunities set forth in paragraphs (b) and (e) above shall be accorded to persons serving on Expert Advisory Panels of the Organization in the exercise of their functions as such.

(iii) Privileges and immunities are granted to the experts of the Organization in the interests of the Organization and not for the personal benefit of the individuals themselves. The Organization shall have the right and the duty to waive the immunity of any expert in any case where in its opinion the immunity would impede the course of justice and it can be waived without prejudice to the interests of the Organization.

3. Article V and Section 25, paragraphs 1 and 2 (I), of Article VII shall extend to the representatives of Associate Members participating in the work of the Organization in accordance with Articles 8 and 47 of the Constitution.

4. The privileges, immunities, exemptions and facilities referred to in Section 21 of the standard clauses shall also be accorded to any Deputy Director-General, Assistant Director-General and Regional Director of the Organization.

---

[1] Adopted by the First World Health Assembly on 17 July 1948 (*Off. Rec. Wld Hlth Org.* **13**, 97, 332) and amended by the Third, Tenth and Eleventh World Health Assemblies (resolutions WHA3.102, WHA10.26 and WHA11.30).

AGREEMENTS
WITH OTHER INTERGOVERNMENTAL
ORGANIZATIONS

AGREEMENT BETWEEN THE WORLD HEALTH
ORGANIZATION AND THE PAN AMERICAN
HEALTH ORGANIZATION[1]

Whereas Chapter XI of the Constitution of the World Health Organization provides that the Pan American Sanitary Organization[2] represented by the Pan American Sanitary Bureau and the Pan American Sanitary Conference shall in due course be integrated with the World Health Organization and that such integration shall be effected as soon as practicable through common action based on mutual consent of the competent authorities expressed through the organizations concerned; and

Whereas the World Health Organization and the Pan American Sanitary Organization have agreed that measures towards the implementation of such action by the conclusion of an agreement shall be taken when at least fourteen American countries shall have ratified the Constitution of the World Health Organization; and

Whereas on the twenty-second of April 1949 this condition was satisfied,

IT IS HEREBY AGREED AS FOLLOWS:

Article 1

The States and territories of the Western Hemisphere make up the geographical area of a regional organization of the World Health Organization, as provided in Chapter XI of its Constitution.

Article 2

The Pan American Sanitary Conference, through the Directing Council of the Pan American Sanitary Organization and the Pan American Sanitary Bureau, shall serve respectively as the Regional Committee and the Regional Office of the World Health Organization for the Western Hemisphere, within the provisions of the Constitution of the World Health Organization. In deference to tradition, both organizations shall retain their

---

[1] Approved by the Second World Health Assembly on 30 June 1949 in resolution WHA2.91.
[2] Renamed "Pan American Health Organization" by decision of the XV Pan American Sanitary Conference, September-October 1958.

respective names, to which shall be added "Regional Committee of the World Health Organization" and "Regional Office of the World Health Organization" respectively.

Article 3

The Pan American Sanitary Conference may adopt and promote health and sanitary conventions and programmes in the Western Hemisphere, provided that such conventions and programmes are compatible with the policy and programmes of the World Health Organization and are separately financed.

Article 4

When this Agreement enters into force, the Director of the Pan American Sanitary Bureau shall assume, subject to the provisions of Article 2, the post of Regional Director of the World Health Organization, until the termination of the period for which he was elected. Thereafter, the Regional Director shall be appointed in accordance with the provisions of Articles 49 and 52 of the World Health Organization Constitution.

Article 5

In accordance with the provisions of Article 51 of the Constitution of the World Health Organization, the Director-General of the World Health Organization shall receive from the Director of the Pan American Sanitary Bureau full information regarding the administration and the operations of the Pan American Sanitary Bureau as the Regional Office for the Western Hemisphere.

Article 6

An adequate proportion of the budget of the World Health Organization shall be allocated for regional work.

Article 7

The annual budget estimates for the expenses of the Pan American Sanitary Bureau as the Regional Office for the Western Hemisphere shall be prepared by the Regional Director and shall be submitted to the Director-General for his consideration in the preparation of the annual budget estimates of the World Health Organization.

Article 8

The funds allocated to the Pan American Sanitary Bureau, as Regional Office of the World Health Organization, under the budget of the World

Health Organization, shall be managed in accordance with the financial policies and procedures of the World Health Organization.

Article 9

This Agreement may be supplemented with the consent of both parties, on the initiative of either party.

Article 10

This Agreement shall enter into force upon its approval by the World Health Assembly and signature by the Director of the Pan American Sanitary Bureau, acting on behalf of the Pan American Sanitary Conference, provided that fourteen of the American Republics have at that time deposited their instruments of acceptance of the Constitution of the World Health Organization.

Article 11

In case of doubt or difficulty in interpretation, the English text shall govern.

IN WITNESS WHEREOF this Agreement was done and signed at Washington on this twenty-fourth day of May nineteen hundred and forty-nine in four copies, two in English and two in French.

For the World Health Organization:	For the Pan American Sanitary Conference:
Brock CHISHOLM, *Director-General*	Fred SOPER, *The Director*

AGREEMENT BETWEEN THE UNITED NATIONS AND THE WORLD HEALTH ORGANIZATION[1]

Preamble

Article 57 of the Charter of the United Nations provides that specialized agencies established by intergovernmental agreement and having wide international responsibilities as defined in their basic instruments in economic, social, cultural, educational, health and related fields shall be brought into relationship with the United Nations.

Article 69 of the Constitution of the World Health Organization provides that the Organization shall be brought into relation with the United Nations as one of the specialized agencies referred to in Article 57 of the Charter.

Therefore, the United Nations and the World Health Organization agree as follows:

Article I

The United Nations recognizes the World Health Organization as the specialized agency responsible for taking such action as may be appropriate under its Constitution for the accomplishment of the objectives set forth therein.

Article II – Reciprocal Representation

1. Representatives of the United Nations shall be invited to attend the meetings of the World Health Assembly and its committees, the Executive Board, and such general, regional or other special meetings as the Organization may convene, and to participate, without vote, in the deliberations of these bodies.

2. Representatives of the World Health Organization shall be invited to attend the meetings of the Economic and Social Council of the United Nations (hereinafter called the Council) and of its commissions and committees, and to participate, without vote, in the deliberations of these bodies with respect to items on their agenda relating to health matters.

3. Representatives of the World Health Organization shall be invited to attend meetings of the General Assembly for purposes of consultation on matters within the scope of its competence.

---

[1] Adopted by the First World Health Assembly on 10 July 1948 (*Off. Rec. Wld Hlth Org.*, **13**, 81, 321).

4. Representatives of the World Health Organization shall be invited to attend meetings of the main committees of the General Assembly when matters within the scope of its competence are under discussion, and to participate, without vote, in such discussions.

5. Representatives of the World Health Organization shall be invited to attend the meetings of the Trusteeship Council, and to participate, without vote, in the deliberations thereof with respect to items on the agenda relating to matters within the competence of the World Health Organization.

6. Written statements of the World Health Organization shall be distributed by the Secretariat of the United Nations to all Members of the General Assembly, the Council and its commissions and the Trusteeship Council as appropriate. Similarly, written statements presented by the United Nations shall be distributed by the World Health Organization to all members of the World Health Assembly or the Executive Board, as appropriate.

Article III – Proposal of Agenda Items

Subject to such preliminary consultation as may be necessary, the World Health Organization shall include on the agenda of the Health Assembly or Executive Board, as appropriate, items proposed to it by the United Nations. Similarly, the Council and its commissions and the Trusteeship Council shall include on their agenda items proposed by the World Health Organization.

Article IV – Recommendations of the United Nations

1. The World Health Organization, having regard to the obligation of the United Nations to promote the objectives set forth in Article 55 of the Charter, and the function and power of the Council, under Article 62 of the Charter, to make or initiate studies and reports with respect to international, economic, social, cultural, educational, health and related matters and to make recommendations concerning these matters to the specialized agencies concerned, and having regard also to the responsibility of the United Nations, under Articles 58 and 63 of the Charter, to make recommendations for the co-ordination of the policies and activities of such specialized agencies, agrees to arrange for the submission, as soon as possible, to the Health Assembly, the Executive Board or such other organ of the World Health Organization as may be appropriate, of all formal recommendations which the United Nations may make to it.

2. The World Health Organization agrees to enter into consultation with the United Nations, upon request, with respect to such recommendations,

and in due course to report to the United Nations on the action taken by the Organization or by its members to give effect to such recommendations, or on the other results of their consideration.

3. The World Health Organization affirms its intention of co-operating in whatever further measures may be necessary to make co-ordination of the activities of specialized agencies and those of the United Nations fully effective. In particular, it agrees to participate in and to co-operate with any body or bodies which the Council may establish for the purpose of facilitating such co-ordination and to furnish such information as may be required for the carrying-out of this purpose.

Article V – Exchange of Information and Documents

1. Subject to such arrangements as may be necessary for the safeguarding of confidential material, the fullest and promptest exchange of information and documents shall be made between the United Nations and the World Health Organization.

2. Without prejudice to the generality of the provisions of paragraph 1:

(a) The World Health Organization agrees to transmit to the United Nations regular reports on the activities of the Organization;

(b) The World Health Organization agrees to comply to the fullest extent practicable with any request which the United Nations may make for the furnishing of special reports, studies or information, subject to the conditions set forth in Article XVI;

(c) The Secretary-General shall, upon request, transmit to the Director-General of the World Health Organization such information, documents or other material as may from time to time be agreed between them.

Article VI – Public Information

Having regard to the functions of the World Health Organization, as defined in Article 2, paragraphs (q) and (r) of its Constitution, to provide information in the field of health and to assist in developing an informed public opinion among all peoples on matters of health, and with a view to furthering co-operation and developing joint services in the field of public information between the Organization and the United Nations, a subsidiary agreement on such matters shall be concluded as soon as possible after the coming-into-force of the present agreement.

Article VII – Assistance to the Security Council

The World Health Organization agrees to co-operate with the Council in furnishing such information and rendering such assistance for the maintenance or restoration of international peace and security as the Security Council may request.

Article VIII – Assistance to the Trusteeship Council

The World Health Organization agrees to co-operate with the Trusteeship Council in the carrying-out of its functions, and in particular agrees that it will, to the greatest extent possible, render such assistance as the Trusteeship Council may request in regard to matters with which the Organization is concerned.

Article IX – Non-self-governing Territories

The World Health Organization agrees to co-operate with the United Nations in giving effect to the principles and obligations set forth in Chapter XI of the Charter with regard to matters affecting the well-being and development of the peoples of non-self-governing territories.

Article X – Relations with the International Court of Justice

1. The World Health Organization agrees to furnish any information which may be requested by the International Court of Justice in pursuance of Article 34 of the Statute of the Court.

2. The General Assembly authorizes the World Health Organization to request advisory opinions of the International Court of Justice on legal questions arising within the scope of its competence other than questions concerning the mutual relationships of the Organization and the United Nations or other specialized agencies.

3. Such requests may be addressed to the Court by the Health Assembly or by the Executive Board acting in pursuance of an authorization by the Health Assembly.

4. When requesting the International Court of Justice to give an advisory opinion, the World Health Organization shall inform the Economic and Social Council of the request.

Article XI – Headquarters and Regional Offices

1. The World Health Organization agrees to consult with the United Nations before making any decision concerning the location of its permanent headquarters.

2. Any regional or branch offices which the World Health Organization may establish shall, so far as practicable, be closely associated with such regional or branch offices as the United Nations may establish.

Article XII – Personnel Arrangements

1. The United Nations and the World Health Organization recognize that the eventual development of a single unified international civil service is desirable from the standpoint of effective administrative co-ordination, and with this end in view agree to develop as far as practicable common personnel standards, methods and arrangements designed to avoid serious discrepancies in terms and conditions of employment, to avoid competition in recruitment of personnel and to facilitate interchange of personnel in order to obtain the maximum benefit from their services.

2. The United Nations and the World Health Organization agree to co-operate to the fullest extent possible in achieving these ends, and in particular they agree to:

(a) Consult together concerning the establishment of an international civil service commission to advise on the means by which common standards of recruitment in the secretariats of the United Nations and of the specialized agencies may be ensured;

(b) Consult together concerning other matters relating to the employment of their officers and staff, including conditions of service, duration of appointments, classification, salary scales and allowances, retirement and pension rights, and staff regulations and rules, with a view to securing as much uniformity in these matters as shall be found practicable;

(c) Co-operate in the interchange of personnel, when desirable, on a temporary or permanent basis, making due provision for the retention of seniority and pension rights;

(d) Co-operate in the establishment and operation of suitable machinery for the settlement of disputes arising in connexion with the employment of personnel and related matters.

Article XIII – Statistical Services

1. The United Nations and the World Health Organization agree to strive for maximum co-operation, the elimination of all undesirable duplication between them, and the most efficient use of their technical personnel in their respective collection, analysis, publication and dissemination of statistical information. They agree to combine their efforts to secure the greatest

possible usefulness and utilization of statistical information and to minimize the burdens placed upon national governments and other organizations from which such information may be collected.

2. The World Health Organization recognizes the United Nations as the central agency for the collection, analysis, publication, standardization, dissemination and improvement of statistics serving the general purposes of international organizations.

3. The United Nations recognizes the World Health Organization as the appropriate agency for the collection, analysis, publication, standardization, dissemination and improvement of statistics within its special sphere, without prejudice to the right of the United Nations to concern itself with such statistics so far as they may be essential for its own purposes or for the improvement of statistics throughout the world.

4. The United Nations shall, in consultation with the specialized agencies, develop administrative instruments and procedures through which effective statistical co-operation may be secured between the United Nations and the agencies brought into relationship with it.

5. It is recognized as desirable that the collection of statistical information should not be duplicated by the United Nations or any of the specialized agencies whenever it is practicable for any of them to utilize information or materials which another may have available.

6. In order to build up a central collection of statistical information for general use, it is agreed that data supplied to the World Health Organization for incorporation in its basic statistical series or special reports should, so far as practicable, be made available to the United Nations.

Article XIV – Administrative and Technical Services

1. The United Nations and the World Health Organization recognize the desirability, in the interest of administrative and technical uniformity and of the most efficient use of personnel and resources, of avoiding, whenever possible, the establishment and operation of competitive or overlapping facilities and services among the United Nations and the specialized agencies.

2. Accordingly, the United Nations and the World Health Organization agree to consult together concerning the establishment and use of common administrative and technical services and facilities, in addition to those referred to in Articles XII, XIII and XV, in so far as the establishment and use of such services may, from time to time, be found practicable and appropriate.

3. Arrangements shall be made between the United Nations and the World Health Organization in regard to the registration and deposit of official documents.

Article XV – Budgetary and Financial Arrangements

1. The World Health Organization recognizes the desirability of establishing close budgetary and financial relationships with the United Nations, in order that the administrative operations of the United Nations and of the specialized agencies shall be carried out in the most efficient and economical manner possible, and that the maximum measure of co-ordination and uniformity with respect to these operations shall be secured.

2. The United Nations and the World Health Organization agree to co-operate to the fullest extent possible in achieving these ends and, in particular, shall consult together concerning the desirability of the inclusion of the budget of the Organization within a general budget of the United Nations. Any arrangements to this effect shall be defined in a supplementary agreement between the two organizations.

3. Pending the conclusion of any such agreement, the following arrangement shall govern budgetary and financial relationships between the World Health Organization and the United Nations:

(*a*) The Secretary-General and the Director-General shall arrange for consultation in connexion with the preparation of the budget of the World Health Organization.

(*b*) The World Health Organization agrees to transmit its proposed budget to the United Nations annually at the same time as such budget is transmitted to its members. The General Assembly shall examine the budget or proposed budget of the Organization and may make recommendations to it concerning any item or items contained therein.

(*c*) Representatives of the World Health Organization shall be entitled to participate, without vote, in the deliberations of the General Assembly or any committee thereof, at all times when the budget of the World Health Organization or general administrative or financial questions affecting the Organization are under consideration.

(*d*) The United Nations may undertake the collection of contributions from those members of the World Health Organization which are also Members of the United Nations, in accordance with such arrangements as may be defined by a later agreement between the United Nations and the Organization.

(*e*) The United Nations shall, upon its own initiative or upon the request of the World Health Organization, arrange for studies to be undertaken concerning other financial and fiscal questions of interest to the Organization and to other specialized agencies, with a view to the provision of common services and the securing of uniformity in such matters.

(*f*) The World Health Organization agrees to conform, as far as may be practicable, to standard practices and forms recommended by the United Nations.

Article XVI – Financing of Special Services

1. In the event of the World Health Organization being faced with the necessity of incurring substantial extra expense as a result of any request which the United Nations may make for special reports, studies or assistance in accordance with Articles V, VII, VIII, or with other provisions of this agreement, consultation shall take place with a view to determining the most equitable manner in which such expense shall be borne.

2. Consultation between the United Nations and the World Health Organization shall similarly take place with a view to making such arrangements as may be found equitable for covering the cost of central administrative, technical or fiscal services or facilities or other special assistance provided by the United Nations, in so far as they apply to the World Health Organization.

Article XVII – Laissez-passer

Officials of the World Health Organization shall have the right to use the *laissez-passer* of the United Nations in accordance with special arrangements to be negotiated between the Secretary-General of the United Nations and the Director-General of the World Health Organization.

Article XVIII – Interagency Agreements

The World Health Organization agrees to inform the Council of any formal agreement between the Organization and any other specialized agency, intergovernmental organization or non-governmental organization and in particular agrees to inform the Council of the nature and scope of any such agreement before it is concluded.

Article XIX – Liaison

1. The United Nations and the World Health Organization agree to the foregoing provisions in the belief that they will contribute to the maintenance of effective liaison between the two organizations. They affirm their

intention of taking whatever further measures may be necessary to make this liaison fully effective.

2. The liaison arrangements provided for in the foregoing articles of this agreement shall apply as far as appropriate to the relations between such branch or regional offices as may be established by the two organizations, as well as between their central headquarters.

Article XX – Implementation of the Agreement

The Secretary-General and the Director-General may enter into such supplementary arrangements for the implementation of this agreement as may be found desirable, in the light of the operating experience of the two organizations.

Article XXI – Revision

This agreement shall be subject to revision by agreement between the United Nations and the World Health Organization.

Article XXII – Entry-into-Force

This agreement shall come into force on its approval by the General Assembly of the United Nations and the World Health Assembly.

AGREEMENT BETWEEN THE INTERNATIONAL LABOUR ORGANISATION AND THE WORLD HEALTH ORGANIZATION[1]

Article I – Co-operation and Consultation

The International Labour Organisation and the World Health Organization agree that, with a view to facilitating the effective attainment of the objectives set forth in their respective Constitutions within the general framework established by the Charter of the United Nations, they will act in close co-operation with each other and will consult each other regularly in regard to matters of common interest.

Article II – Reciprocal Representation

1. Representatives of the International Labour Organisation shall be invited to attend the meetings of the Executive Board of the World Health Organization and the World Health Assembly and to participate without vote in the deliberations of each of these bodies and of their commissions and committees with respect to items on their agenda in which the International Labour Organisation has an interest.

2. Representatives of the World Health Organization shall be invited to attend the meetings of the Governing Body of the International Labour Office and the International Labour Conference and to participate without vote in the deliberations of each of these bodies and of their committees with respect to items on their agenda in which the World Health Organization has an interest.

3. Appropriate arrangements shall be made by agreement from time to time for the reciprocal representation of the International Labour Organisation and the World Health Organization at other meetings convened under their respective auspices which consider matters in which the other organization has an interest.

Article III – ILO/WHO Joint Committees

1. The International Labour Organisation and the World Health Organization may refer to a joint committee any question of common interest which it may appear desirable to refer to such a committee.

---

[1] Adopted by the First World Health Assembly on 10 July 1948 (*Off. Rec. Wld Hlth Org.*, **13**, 81, 322): see also resolution WHA2.101.

2. Any such joint committee shall consist of representatives appointed by each organization, the number to be appointed by each being decided by agreement between the two organizations.

3. The United Nations shall be invited to designate a representative to attend the meetings of any such joint committee; the committee may also invite other specialized agencies to be represented at its meetings as may be found desirable.

4. The reports of any such joint committee shall be communicated to the Director-General of each organization for submission to the appropriate body or bodies of the two organizations; a copy of the reports of the committee shall be communicated to the Secretary-General of the United Nations for the information of the Economic and Social Council.

5. Any such joint committee shall regulate its own procedure.

Article IV – Exchange of Information and Documents

1. Subject to such arrangements as may be necessary for the safeguarding of confidential material, the fullest and promptest exchange of information and documents shall be made between the International Labour Organisation and the World Health Organization.

2. The Director-General of the International Labour Office and the Director-General of the World Health Organization, or their authorized representatives, shall, upon the request of either party, consult with each other regarding the provision by either organization of such information as may be of interest to the other.

Article V – Personnel Arrangements

The International Labour Organisation and the World Health Organization agree that the measures to be taken by them, within the framework of the general arrangements for co-operation in regard to staff personnel to be made by the United Nations, will include:

(a) Measures to avoid competition in the recruitment of their personnel; and

(b) Measures to facilitate interchange of personnel on a temporary or permanent basis, in appropriate cases, in order to obtain the maximum benefit from their services, making due provision for the retention of seniority and pension rights.

Article VI – Statistical Services

1. The International Labour Organisation and the World Health Organization agree to strive, within the framework of the general arrangements for

statistical co-operation made by the United Nations, for maximum co-operation with a view to the most efficient use of their technical personnel in their respective collection, analysis, publication, standardization, improvement and dissemination of statistical information. They recognize the desirability of avoiding duplication in the collection of statistical information whenever it is practicable for either of them to utilize information or materials which the other may have available or may be specially qualified and prepared to collect, and agree to combine their efforts to secure the greatest possible usefulness and utilization of statistical information, and to minimize the burdens placed upon national governments and other organizations from which such information may be collected.

2. The International Labour Organisation and the World Health Organization agree to keep each other informed of their work in the field of statistics and to consult each other in regard to all statistical projects dealing with matters of common interest.

Article VII – Financing of Special Services

If compliance with a request for assistance made by either organization to the other would involve substantial expenditure for the organization complying with the request, consultation shall take place with a view to determining the most equitable manner of meeting such expenditure.

Article VIII – Implementation of the Agreement

1. The Director-General of the International Labour Office and the Director-General of the World Health Organization may enter into such supplementary arrangements for the implementation of this agreement as may be found desirable in the light of the operating experience of the two organizations.

2. The liaison arrangements provided for in the foregoing articles of this agreement shall apply as far as appropriate to the relations between such branch or regional offices as may be established by the two organizations as well as between their central machinery.

Article IX – Notification to and Registration by the United Nations

1. In accordance with their respective agreements with the United Nations, the International Labour Organisation and the World Health Organization will inform the Economic and Social Council forthwith of the terms of the present agreement.

2. On the coming-into-force of the present agreement, in accordance with the provisions of Article XI, it will be communicated to the Secretary-General of the United Nations for filing and recording, in pursuance of Article 10 of the Regulations, to give effect to Article 102 of the Charter of the United Nations adopted by the General Assembly of the United Nations on 14 December 1946.

Article X – Revision and Termination

1. This agreement shall be subject to revision by agreement between the International Labour Organisation and the World Health Organization and shall be reviewed in any case not later than three years after the agreement has come into force.

2. If agreement on the subject of revision cannot be reached, the agreement may be terminated by either party on 31 December of any year by notice to the other party not later than 30 September of that year.

Article XI – Entry-into-Force

This agreement shall come into force on its approval by the Governing Body of the International Labour Office and by the World Health Assembly.

AGREEMENT BETWEEN THE FOOD AND AGRICULTURE ORGANIZATION OF THE UNITED NATIONS AND THE WORLD HEALTH ORGANIZATION[1]

Article I   Co-operation and Consultation

The Food and Agriculture Organization of the United Nations and the World Health Organization agree that, with a view to facilitating the effective attainment of the objectives set forth in their respective Constitutions within the general framework established by the Charter of the United Nations, they will act in close co-operation with each other, and will consult each other regularly in regard to matters of common interest.

Article II – Reciprocal Representation

1. Representatives of FAO shall be invited to attend the meetings of the Executive Board of WHO and of the World Health Assembly and to participate without vote in the deliberations of each of these bodies and of their commissions and committees with respect to items on their agenda in which FAO has an interest.

2. Representatives of WHO shall be invited to attend the meetings of the Executive Committee of FAO, or its successor, and the Conference of FAO and to participate without vote in the deliberations of each of these bodies and of their commissions and committees with respect to items on their agenda in which WHO has an interest.

3. Appropriate arrangements shall be made by agreement from time to time for the reciprocal representation of FAO and WHO at other meetings convened under their respective auspices which consider matters in which the other organization has an interest.

Article III – FAO/WHO Joint Committees

1. FAO and WHO may refer to a joint committee any question of common interest which it may appear desirable to refer to such a committee.

2. Any such joint committee shall consist of representatives appointed by each organization, the number to be appointed by each being decided by agreement between the two organizations.

3. Representatives of the United Nations and of other specialized agen-

---

[1] Adopted by the First World Health Assembly on 17 July 1948 (*Off. Rec. Wld Hlth Org.*, **13**, 96, 323).

cies of the United Nations will be invited to attend the meetings of joint committees and to participate without vote in their deliberations.

4. The reports of any such joint committee shall be communicated to the Director-General of each organization for submission to the appropriate body or bodies of the two organizations.

5. Any such joint committee shall regulate its own internal procedure.

6. Arrangements for the provision of suitable secretariat services for any such joint committee shall be made by agreement between the Director-General of FAO and the Director-General of WHO, or their representatives.

Article IV – FAO/WHO Joint Missions

FAO and WHO may establish joint missions under similar arrangements and procedure to those set forth in Article III.

Article V – Exchange of Information and Documents

1. The Director-General of each organization shall keep the other organization fully informed concerning all programmes of work and projected activities in which there may be mutual interest.

2. Subject to such arrangements as may be necessary for the safeguarding of confidential material, the fullest and promptest exchange of information and documents shall be made between FAO and WHO.

3. The Director-General of FAO and the Director-General of WHO, or their representatives, shall, upon the request of either party, consult with each other regarding the provision by either organization of such special information as may be of interest to the other.

Article VI – Inter-secretariat Committees

The Directors-General of the two organizations, or their representatives, may, when they consider it desirable, establish by agreement inter-secretariat committees to facilitate co-operation in connexion with specific programmes of work or projected activities with which the two organizations may be mutually concerned.

Article VII – Personnel Arrangements

FAO and WHO agree that the measures to be taken by them, within the framework of the general arrangements for co-operation in regard to staff personnel to be made by the United Nations, will include:

(a) Measures to avoid competition in the recruitment of their staff person-

nel, including prior consultation concerning appointments in the technical fields with which both organizations are concerned: and

(*b*) Measures to facilitate interchange of personnel on a temporary or permanent basis, in appropriate cases, in order to obtain the maximum
benefit from their services, making due provision for the retention of
seniority and pension rights.

Article VIII – Statistical Services

1. FAO and WHO agree to strive, within the framework of the general
arrangements for statistical co-operation made by the United Nations, for
maximum co-operation with a view to the most efficient use of their technical personnel in their respective collection, analysis, publication, standardization, improvement and dissemination of statistical information. They
recognize the desirability of avoiding duplication in the collection of statistical information whenever it is practicable for either of them to utilize
information or materials which the other may have available or may be
especially qualified and prepared to collect, and agree to combine their
efforts to secure the greatest possible usefulness and utilization of statistical
information, and to minimize the burdens placed upon national governments and other organizations from which such information may be collected.

2. FAO and WHO agree to keep each other informed of their work in the
field of statistics and to consult each other in regard to all statistical projects
dealing with matters of common interest.

Article IX – Financing of Special Services

If compliance with a request for assistance made by either organization
to the other involves or would involve substantial expenditure for the organization complying with the request, consultation shall take place with a
view to determining the most equitable manner of meeting such expenditure.

Article X – Regional and Branch Offices

FAO and WHO agree to keep each other informed of plans for the initial
establishment and relocation of regional and branch offices and to consult
together with a view, where practicable, to entering into co-operative
arrangements as to location, staffing and the use of common services.

Article XI – Implementation of the Agreement

The Director-General of FAO and the Director-General of WHO shall enter into such supplementary arrangements for the implementation of this agreement as may be found desirable in the light of the operating experience of the two organizations.

*Article XII – Notification to and Registration
by the United Nations*

1. In accordance with their respective agreements with the United Nations, FAO and WHO will inform the Economic and Social Council forthwith of the terms of the present agreement.

2. On the coming-into-force of the present agreement, in accordance with the provisions of Article XIV, it will be communicated to the Secretary-General of the United Nations for filing and recording, in pursuance of Article 10 of the Regulations, to give effect to Article 102 of the Charter of the United Nations, adopted by the General Assembly of the United Nations on 14 December 1946.

Article XIII – Revision and Review

This agreement shall be subject to revision by agreement between FAO and WHO, and shall be reviewed in any case not later than three years after the agreement has come into force.

Article XIV – Entry-into-Force

This agreement shall come into force on its approval by the Conference of FAO and by the World Health Assembly.

AGREEMENT BETWEEN THE UNITED NATIONS EDUCATIONAL, SCIENTIFIC AND CULTURAL ORGANIZATION AND THE WORLD HEALTH ORGANIZATION[1]

Article I – Co-operation and Consultation

1. The World Health Organization and the United Nations Educational, Scientific and Cultural Organization agree that, with a view to facilitating the effective attainment of the objectives set forth in their respective Constitutions within the general framework established by the Charter of the United Nations, they will act in close co-operation with each other and will consult each other regularly in regard to matters of common interest.

2. In particular, it is recognized by UNESCO that WHO shall have the primary responsibility for the encouragement of research, education, and the organization of science in the fields of health and medicine, without prejudice to the right of UNESCO to concern itself with the relations between the pure and applied sciences in all fields, including the sciences basic to health.

3. In case of doubt as to the division of responsibility between the two organizations concerning any projected activity or programme of work, the organization initiating such activity or programme shall consult the other with a view to adjusting the matter by mutual agreement, either by referring it to an appropriate joint committee as provided in Article IV or by other means.

Article II – Reciprocal Representation

1. Representatives of WHO shall be invited to attend the meetings of the Executive Board and General Conference of UNESCO and to participate without vote in the deliberations of these bodies and of their commissions and committees with respect to items on their agenda in which WHO has an interest.

2. Representatives of UNESCO shall be invited to attend the meetings of the Executive Board of WHO and the World Health Assembly and to participate without vote in the deliberations of these bodies and of their commissions and committees with respect to items on their agenda in which UNESCO has an interest.

---

[1] Adopted by the First World Health Assembly on 17 July 1948 (*Off. Rec. Wld Hlth Org.*, **13**, 96, 323).

3. Appropriate arrangements shall be made by agreement between the Directors-General of the two organizations, or their representatives, for the reciprocal representation of WHO and UNESCO at other meetings convened under their respective auspices which consider matters in which the other organization has an interest.

Article III – Proposal of Agenda Items

After such preliminary consultation as may be necessary, each organization shall include in the agenda of the meetings referred to in Article II any question which has been submitted to it by the other organization.

Article IV – UNESCO/WHO Joint Committees

1. UNESCO and WHO may refer to a joint committee any question of common interest which it may appear desirable to refer to such a committee.

2. Any such joint committee shall consist of representatives appointed by each organization, the number to be appointed by each being decided by agreement between the two organizations.

3. The United Nations shall be invited to designate a representative to attend the meetings of any such joint committee; the committee may also invite other specialized agencies to be represented at its meetings as may be found desirable.

4. The reports of each such joint committee shall be communicated to the Director-General of each organization for submission to the appropriate body or bodies of the two organizations; a copy of all such reports shall be communicated to the Secretary-General of the United Nations for the information of the Economic and Social Council.

5. Any such joint committee shall regulate its own procedure.

6. Arrangements for the provision of suitable secretariat services for any joint committee shall be made by agreement between the Directors-General of the two organizations, or their representatives.

Article V – Exchange of Information and Documents

1. The Secretariat of each organization agrees to keep the other fully informed concerning all projected activities and programmes of work in which there may be mutual interest.

2. Subject to such arrangements as may be necessary for the safeguarding of confidential material, the fullest and promptest exchange of information and documents shall be made between WHO and UNESCO.

3. The Director-General of WHO and the Director-General of UNESCO, or their representatives, shall, upon the request of either party, consult each other regarding the provision by either organization of such special information as may be of interest to the other.

Article VI – Personnel Arrangements

WHO and UNESCO agree that the measures to be taken by them, within the framework of the general arrangements for co-operation in regard to personnel matters to be made by the United Nations, will include:

(*a*) Measures to avoid competition in the recruitment of their staff personnel; and

(*b*) Measures to facilitate interchange of personnel on a temporary or permanent basis, in appropriate cases, in order to obtain the maximum benefit from their services, with provision for the protection of seniority and pension rights.

Article VII – Statistical Services

1. WHO and UNESCO agree to strive, within the framework of the general arrangements for statistical co-operation made by the United Nations, for maximum co-operation with a view to the most efficient use of their technical personnel in their respective collection, analysis, publication, standardization, improvement and dissemination of statistical information. Both organizations recognize the desirability of avoiding duplication in the collection of statistical information whenever it is practicable for either of them to utilize information, materials or raw data which the other may have available or may be specifically qualified and prepared to collect, and agree to combine their efforts to secure the greatest possible usefulness and utilization of statistical information, and to minimize the burdens placed upon national governments and other organizations from which such information may be collected.

2. WHO and UNESCO agree to keep each other informed of their work in the field of statistics and to consult each other in regard to all statistical projects dealing with matters of common interest.

Article VIII – Financing of Special Services

If compliance with a request for assistance made by either organization to the other involves or would involve substantial expenditure for the organization complying with the request, consultation shall take place with a view to determining the most equitable manner of meeting such expenditure.

Article IX – Regional and Branch Offices

WHO and UNESCO agree to keep each other informed of plans for the establishment and relocation of regional and branch offices and to consult together with a view, where practicable, to entering into co-operative arrangements as to the premises, staffing and common services.

Article X – Implementation of the Agreement

The Director-General of WHO and the Director-General of UNESCO shall enter into such supplementary arrangements for the implementation of this agreement as may be found desirable in the light of operating experience.

Article XI – Notification to and Registration by the United Nations

1. In accordance with their respective agreements with the United Nations, WHO and UNESCO will inform the Economic and Social Council forthwith of the terms of the present agreement.

2. On the coming-into-force of the present agreement, it will be communicated to the Secretary-General of the United Nations for filing and recording, in pursuance of Article 10 of the Regulations, to give effect to Article 102 of the Charter of the United Nations adopted by the General Assembly on 14 December 1946.

Article XII – Revision and Review

1. This agreement shall be subject to revision by agreement between WHO and UNESCO and shall be reviewed in any case not later than three years after its entry-into-force.

2. If agreement on the subject of revision cannot be reached, the agreement may be terminated by either party on 31 December of any year by notice given to the other party not later than 30 September of that year.

Article XIII – Entry-into-Force

This agreement shall come into force on its approval by the World Health Assembly and by the Executive Board of UNESCO.

AGREEMENT BETWEEN THE INTERNATIONAL ATOMIC ENERGY AGENCY AND THE WORLD HEALTH ORGANIZATION[1]

Article I – Co-operation and Consultation

1. The International Atomic Energy Agency and the World Health Organization agree that, with a view to facilitating the effective attainment of the objectives set forth in their respective constitutional instruments, within the general framework established by the Charter of the United Nations, they will act in close co-operation with each other and will consult each other regularly in regard to matters of common interest.

2. In particular, and in accordance with the Constitution of the World Health Organization and the Statute of the International Atomic Energy Agency and its agreement with the United Nations together with the exchange of letters related thereto, and taking into account the respective co-ordinating responsibilities of both organizations, it is recognized by the World Health Organization that the International Atomic Energy Agency has the primary responsibility for encouraging, assisting and co-ordinating research on, and development and practical application of, atomic energy for peaceful uses throughout the world without prejudice to the right of the World Health Organization to concern itself with promoting, developing, assisting, and co-ordinating international health work, including research, in all its aspects.

3. Whenever either organization proposes to initiate a programme or activity on a subject in which the other organization has or may have a substantial interest, the first party shall consult the other with a view to adjusting the matter by mutual agreement.

Article II – Reciprocal Representation

1. Representatives of the World Health Organization shall be invited to attend the General Conference of the International Atomic Energy Agency and to participate without vote in the deliberations of that body and of its subsidiary organs (e.g. commissions and committees) with respect to items on their agenda in which the World Health Organization has an interest.

2. Representatives of the International Atomic Energy Agency shall be invited to attend the World Health Assembly and to participate without vote

---

[1] Approved by the Twelfth World Health Assembly on 28 May 1959 in resolution WHA12.40.

in the deliberations of that body and of its subsidiary organs (e.g. commissions and committees) with respect to items on their agenda in which the International Atomic Energy Agency has an interest.

3. Representatives of the World Health Organization shall be invited as appropriate to attend meetings of the Board of Governors of the International Atomic Energy Agency and to participate without vote in the deliberations of that body and of its commissions and committees with respect to items on their agenda in which the World Health Organization has an interest.

4. Representatives of the International Atomic Energy Agency shall be invited as appropriate to attend meetings of the Executive Board of the World Health Organization and to participate without vote in the deliberations of that body and of its commissions and committees with respect to items on their agenda in which the International Atomic Energy Agency has an interest.

5. Appropriate arrangements shall be made by agreement from time to time for the reciprocal representation of the International Atomic Energy Agency and the World Health Organization at other meetings convened under their respective auspices which consider matters in which the other organization has an interest.

Article III – Exchange of Information and Documents

1. The International Atomic Energy Agency and the World Health Organization recognize that they may find it necessary to apply certain limitations for the safeguarding of confidential information furnished to them. They therefore agree that nothing in this agreement shall be construed as requiring either of them to furnish such information as would, in the judgement of the party possessing the information, constitute a violation of the confidence of any of its Members or anyone from whom it has received such information or otherwise interfere with the orderly conduct of its operations.

2. Subject to such arrangements as may be necessary for the safeguarding of confidential material, the Secretariat of the International Atomic Energy Agency and the Secretariat of the World Health Organization shall keep each other fully informed concerning all projected activities and all programmes of work which may be of interest to both parties.

3. The Director-General of the World Health Organization and the Director-General of the International Atomic Energy Agency or their representatives shall, at the request of either party, arrange for consultations

regarding the provision by either party of such special information as may be of interest to the other party.

Article IV – Proposal of Agenda Items

After such preliminary consultations as may be necessary, the World Health Organization shall include on the provisional agenda of its Assembly or its Executive Board items proposed to it by the International Atomic Energy Agency. Similarly, the International Atomic Energy Agency shall include on the provisional agenda of its General Conference or its Board of Governors items proposed by the World Health Organization. Items submitted by either party for consideration by the other shall be accompanied by an explanatory memorandum.

Article V – Co-operation between Secretariats

The Secretariat of the International Atomic Energy Agency and the Secretariat of the World Health Organization shall maintain a close working relationship in accordance with such arrangements as may have been agreed upon from time to time between the Directors-General of both organizations. In particular, joint committees may be convened when appropriate to consider questions of substantive interest to both parties.

Article VI – Technical and Administrative Co-operation

1. The International Atomic Energy Agency and the World Health Organization agree to consult each other from time to time regarding the most efficient use of personnel and resources and appropriate methods of avoiding the establishment and operation of competitive or overlapping facilities and services.

2. The International Atomic Energy Agency and the World Health Organization agree that the measures to be taken by them, within the framework of any general arrangements for co-operating in regard to personnel matters which are made by the United Nations, will include

(*a*) measures to avoid competition in the recruitment of their personnel; and

(*b*) measures to facilitate interchange of personnel on a temporary or permanent basis, in appropriate cases, in order to obtain the maximum benefit from their services, making due provision for the protection of the seniority, pension and other rights of the personnel concerned.

Article VII – Statistical Services

In view of the desirability of maximum co-operation in the statistical field and of minimizing the burdens placed on national governments and other organizations from which information may be collected, the International Atomic Energy Agency and the World Health Organization undertake, bearing in mind the general arrangements for statistical co-operation made by the United Nations, to avoid undesirable duplication between them with respect to the collection, compilation and publication of statistics, to consult with each other on the most efficient use of information, resources, and technical personnel in the field of statistics and in regard to all statistical projects dealing with matters of common interest.

Article VIII – Financing of Special Services

If compliance with a request for assistance made by either organization to the other involves or would involve substantial expenditure for the organization complying with the request, consultation shall take place with a view to determining the most equitable manner of meeting such expenditure.

Article IX – Regional and Branch Offices

The World Health Organization and the International Atomic Energy Agency agree to consult together with a view, where practicable, to entering into co-operative arrangements as to the use by either organization of the premises, staffing and common services of regional and branch offices which the other has already established or may establish later.

Article X – Implementation of the Agreement

The Director-General of the International Atomic Energy Agency and the Director-General of the World Health Organization may enter into such arrangements for the implementation of this agreement as may be found desirable in the light of the operating experience of the two organizations.

Article XI – Notification to the United Nations
and Filing and Recording

1. In accordance with their respective agreements with the United Nations, the International Atomic Energy Agency and the World Health Organization will inform the United Nations forthwith of the terms of the present agreement.

2. On the coming-into-force of this agreement it will be submitted to the Secretary-General of the United Nations for filing and recording in accordance with the existing regulations of the United Nations.

Article XII – Revision and Termination

1. This agreement shall be subject to revision by agreement between the World Health Organization and the International Atomic Energy Agency on the request of either party.

2. If agreement on the subject of revision cannot be reached, the agreement may be terminated by either party on 31 December of any year by notice given to the other party not later than 30 June of that year.

Article XIII – Entry-into-Force

This agreement shall come into force on its approval by the General Conference of the International Atomic Energy Agency and by the World Health Assembly.

AGREEMENT BETWEEN THE INTERNATIONAL FUND FOR AGRICULTURAL DEVELOPMENT AND THE WORLD HEALTH ORGANIZATION[1]

WHEREAS the World Health Organization (hereinafter referred to as "WHO") and the International Fund for Agricultural Development (hereinafter referred to as "IFAD") have common interest in the well-being and health of the people in their Member countries, especially in the developing Member countries,

WHEREAS both organizations desire to cooperate with each other in order to achieve their common objectives,

WHEREAS Article 2(*b*) of the Constitution of WHO provides *inter alia* that the Organization shall establish and maintain effective collaboration with the United Nations and its specialized agencies,

WHEREAS Article 8, section 2, of the agreement establishing IFAD provides that IFAD shall cooperate closely with the organizations of the United Nations system,

WHO AND IFAD HAVE AGREED AS FOLLOWS:

Article I – Competence of the Two Parties

1.1 WHO recognizes IFAD's special role in mobilizing additional resources to be made available on concessional terms for agricultural development in its developing Member countries primarily for projects and programmes specifically designed to introduce, expand or improve food production systems and to strengthen related policies and institutions within the framework of national priorities and strategies, taking into consideration: the need to increase food production in the poorest food deficit countries; the potential for increasing food production in other developing countries; and the importance of improving the nutritional level of the poorest populations in developing countries and the conditions of their lives.

1.2 IFAD recognizes WHO's special role in international health work, in particular in such fields as health of rural people, improvement of nutrition and control of communicable diseases.

---

[1] Approved by the Thirty-third World Health Assembly on 23 May 1980 in resolution WHA33.21.

Article II – Consultation and Cooperation

2.1 WHO and IFAD agree to keep each other regularly informed about their respective activities of mutual interest in the area of agricultural development, especially in their common developing Member countries.

2.2 WHO shall endeavour to bring to the attention of IFAD such programmes and projects as may *prima facie* be suitable for assistance from IFAD, and to the extent possible IFAD shall keep WHO informed about the suitability of such programmes and projects for assistance from IFAD.

2.3 Any activity in which the two parties cooperate shall be carried out in conformity with the policies and regulations of the two organizations.

Article III – Areas of Cooperation

3.1 Without prejudice to cooperation in additional fields the two parties agree to consider the following activities as potential fields for mutual cooperation:

3.1.1 programmes and projects designed to increase food production with the improvement of the nutritional status as an essential component, particularly among rural populations;

3.1.2 promotion of appropriate environmental health measures and safeguards as part of agricultural development projects, including the prevention and control of waterborne and other communicable diseases which may be facilitated by irrigation and other agricultural development projects;

3.1.3 rural development programmes which include the improvement of health conditions and community water supply as integral elements.

Article IV – Methods of Cooperation

4.1 Subject to such arrangements as may be necessary to safeguard the confidentiality of any information or document, WHO and IFAD shall provide each other with all such data, documents and information as may be necessary for any activity to be carried out under this agreement.

4.2 The two parties shall, to the extent they deem desirable by mutual consent, provide assistance to each other in studies in the fields of mutual concern.

4.3 IFAD shall whenever it deems appropriate request WHO to assist IFAD in the missions related to its operational activities, with a view to ensuring and facilitating as may be relevant collaboration between the two parties in the planning, implementation and evaluation stages of projects of mutual interest to the two parties.

4.4 WHO and IFAD shall cooperate fully on terms and conditions satisfactory to each other. IFAD, in carrying out its functions, shall make use, as it deems appropriate, of the services and expertise of WHO.

Article V – Administrative Arrangements

5.1 WHO and IFAD shall cooperate to make arrangements they deem necessary for efficient contacts at the technical and coordination level, including as required visits by staff members to the respective headquarters and regional offices.

Article VI – Reciprocal Representation

6.1 WHO shall invite IFAD to be represented at sessions of the World Health Assembly, and such other meetings held under the auspices of WHO as are of interest to IFAD, and to participate without the right to vote in their deliberations on items on their agenda in which IFAD has an interest.

6.2 IFAD shall invite WHO to be represented at meetings of its Governing Council, and such other meetings held under the auspices of IFAD which are not restricted to statutory membership and are of interest to WHO, and to participate without the right to vote in their deliberations on items on their agenda in which WHO has an interest.

Article VII – Financial Arrangements

7.1 IFAD shall reimburse WHO for all the direct staff costs and any additional indirect costs, for example, travel and per diem for services performed by WHO at the specific request of IFAD, and in accordance with financial arrangements to be agreed upon between the two parties.

Article VIII – Final Provisions

8.1 This Agreement shall enter into force on the date on which it is signed by the duly authorized representatives of WHO and IFAD.

8.2 This Agreement may be modified with the consent of the two parties in accordance with their respective constitutional procedures.

8.3 This Agreement may be terminated by mutual agreement, or may be denounced by either party giving the other party six months' written notice. Notwithstanding the expiry of a notice of termination, the two parties agree that the provisions of this Agreement shall remain in full force to the extent necessary to permit the orderly conclusion of any activity undertaken pursuant to this Agreement.

8.4 The Director-General of WHO and the President of IFAD may enter into such supplementary arrangements within the scope of this Agreement as may be desirable in the light of the operating experience of the two organizations to implement this Agreement.

IN FAITH WHEREOF the President of the International Fund for Agricultural Development and the Director-General of the World Health Organization have signed the present Agreement in two copies, in French and English, both texts being equally authentic.

International Fund for Agricultural Development	World Health Organization
Abdelmuhsin M. AL-SUDEARY President	H. MAHLER, M.D. Director-General

AGREEMENT BETWEEN THE UNITED NATIONS INDUSTRIAL DEVELOPMENT ORGANIZATION AND THE WORLD HEALTH ORGANIZATION[1]

Article 1 – Co-operation and Consultation

With a view to facilitating the effective attainment of the objectives set forth in their respective Constitutions, the United Nations Industrial Development Organization (hereinafter referred to as "UNIDO") and the World Health Organization (hereinafter referred to as "WHO") agree that, within the general framework established by the Charter of the United Nations and by their respective Constitutions, they shall act in close co-operation with each other and they shall consult with each other regularly in regard to matters of common interest.

Article 2 – Reciprocal Representation

1. Representatives of WHO shall be invited to attend the sessions of the General Conference and of the Industrial Development Board of UNIDO and to participate without vote in the deliberations of each of these bodies on matters of particular concern to WHO.

2. Representatives of UNIDO shall be invited to attend the sessions of the Executive Board of WHO and the World Health Assembly and to participate without vote in the deliberations of each of these bodies on matters of particular concern to UNIDO.

Article 3 – Proposal of Agenda Items

Upon request by the other organization, and after such preliminary consultations as may be necessary, each organization shall include in the provisional agenda of the session respectively referred to in Article 2, paragraphs 1 and 2, any question which has been submitted to it by the other organization.

Article 4 – Exchange of Information and Documents

Subject to such arrangements as may be necessary for the safeguarding of confidential material, the fullest and promptest exchange of information

---

[1] Approved by the Forty-second World Health Assembly on 19 May 1989 in resolution WHA42.21.

and documentation shall be made between UNIDO and WHO. The information so provided shall in particular cover all projected activities and all programmes of work which may be of interest to the other party.

Article 5 – Co-operation between Secretariats

The Secretariat of UNIDO and the Secretariat of WHO shall maintain a close working relationship in accordance with such arrangements as may have been agreed upon from time to time between the Directors-General of UNIDO and WHO.

Article 6 – UNIDO/WHO Joint Committees

1. UNIDO and WHO may refer to a joint committee any questions of common interest which it may appear desirable to refer to such a committee.

2. Any such joint committee shall consist of representatives appointed by each organization, the number to be appointed by each being decided by agreement between the two organizations.

Article 7 – Statistical Services

UNIDO and WHO agree to keep each other informed of their work in the field of statistics and to consult each other in regard to all statistical projects dealing with matters of common interest.

Article 8 – Personnel Arrangements

WHO and UNIDO agree to co-operate in order to facilitate the interchange of staff and to promote efficiency and effective co-ordination on their respective activities. Such co-operation shall be in accordance with the Inter-Organization Agreement Concerning Transfer, Secondment or Loan of Staff among the Organizations Applying the United Nations Common System of Salaries and Allowances.

Article 9 – Financing of Special Services

If compliance with a request for assistance made by either organization to the other would involve substantial expenditure for the organization complying with the request, consultation shall take place with a view to determining the most equitable manner of meeting such expenditure.

Article 10 – Implementation of the Agreement

The Directors-General of UNIDO and WHO may enter into such arrangements for the implementation of this Agreement as may be found desirable in the light of the operating experience of the two organizations.

Article 11 – Notification to the United Nations and Filing and Recording

1. In accordance with their respective agreements with the United Nations, UNIDO and WHO shall inform the United Nations forthwith of the terms of the present Agreement.

2. On the coming-into-force of the present Agreement in accordance with the provisions of Article 13, it shall be communicated to the Secretary-General of the United Nations for filing and recording.

Article 12 – Revision and Termination

1. This Agreement shall be subject to revision by agreement between UNIDO and WHO.

2. It may be terminated by either party on 31 December of any year by written notice given not later than 30 June of that year.

Article 13 – Entry-into-Force

This Agreement shall enter into force upon having been approved by the Industrial Development Board of UNIDO and the World Health Assembly of WHO and signed by the Directors-General of UNIDO and WHO, respectively.

AGREEMENT BETWEEN THE WORLD HEALTH ORGANIZATION AND THE UNIVERSAL POSTAL UNION [1]

Preamble

The World Health Organization (hereinafter referred to as WHO) and the Universal Postal Union (hereinafter referred to as the UPU),

Wishing to coordinate their efforts within the framework of the missions assigned to them,

Recognizing that the WHO is the United Nations specialized agency responsible for providing information, counsel, and assistance in the field of health; promoting cooperation among scientific and professional groups which contribute to the advancement of health; and advancing work in the prevention and control of the international spread of diseases,

Recognizing that the UPU is the United Nations specialized agency the purpose of which is to organize and improve the postal services and to promote, in this field, the safe transport of mail,

Recognizing the desirability of the UPU's cooperating, within the field of its competence, with WHO in promoting, among other things:

a   the safe transport of infectious substances;

b   the safe transport of diagnostic specimens;

c   the development of safer packaging systems at minimum cost;

d   the development of simple labelling to aid compliance;

e   the development of training programmes and awareness campaigns to introduce recommendations in all countries,

Have agreed on the following:

Article I – Mutual consultation

1   WHO and the UPU shall consult as needed on policy issues and matters of common interest for the purpose of realizing their objectives and coordinating their respective activities.

2   WHO and the UPU shall exchange information on developments in any of their fields and projects that are of mutual interest and shall reciprocally

---

[1]   Approved by the Fifty-second World Health Assembly on 24 May 1999 in resolution WHA52.6.

take observations concerning such activities into consideration with a view to promoting effective coordination.

3 When appropriate, consultations shall be arranged at the required level between representatives of the UPU and WHO to agree upon the most effective way in which to organize particular activities and to optimize the use of their resources in compliance with their respective mandates.

Article II – Exchange of information

1 WHO and the UPU shall combine their efforts to achieve the best use of all available information relevant to the transportation of infectious substances using the postal services.

Article III – Reciprocal representation

1 Appropriate arrangements may be made for the reciprocal representation at WHO and UPU meetings convened under their respective auspices and which consider matters in which the other party has an interest or technical competence.

2 The Director-General of the International Bureau of the UPU and the Director-General of WHO shall appoint a focal point with a view to ensuring the implementation of the provisions of the present Agreement.

Article IV – Technical cooperation

1 When in the interest of their respective activities, WHO and the UPU shall seek each other's expertise to optimize the effects of such activities.

2 The UPU shall endeavour, through its bodies as well as its Postal Security Action Group (PSAG), to sensitize the national postal administrations to the need to apply measures to ensure the safe transport of infectious substances.

3 By mutual agreement, the UPU and WHO shall associate themselves in the development and execution of programmes, projects and activities relating particularly to the safe transport of infectious substances through the post.

4 Joint activities to be conducted under the present Agreement shall be subject to the approval of individual project documents by both parties and shall be monitored under an agreed mechanism.

5 WHO and the UPU shall cooperate in evaluating such programmes, projects and activities as have common interest subject to mutual agreement on a case-by-case basis.

Article V – Entry into force, modification and duration

1 The present Agreement shall enter into force on the date on which it is signed by the Director-General of WHO and the Director-General of the International Bureau of the UPU, subject to the approval of the UPU Council of Administration and the World Health Assembly.

2 The Agreement may be modified by mutual consent expressed in writing. It may also be revoked by either party by giving six months' notice to the other party.

In witness whereof, the Director-General of the World Health Organization and the Director-General of the International Bureau of the Universal Postal Union sign the present Agreement in duplicate, in English and French, both texts being authentic, on the dates appearing under their respective signatures.

AGREEMENT BETWEEN
THE OFFICE INTERNATIONAL DES ÉPIZOOTIES AND
THE WORLD HEALTH ORGANIZATION[1]

The World Health Organization (hereinafter referred to as WHO) and the Office International des Épizooties (hereinafter referred to as the OIE) wishing to co-ordinate their efforts for the promotion and improvement of veterinary public health (VPH) and food security and safety, and to collaborate closely for this purpose

Have agreed to the following:

Article 1

1.1   WHO and the OIE agree to cooperate closely in matters of common interest pertaining to their respective fields of competence as defined by their respective constitutional instruments and by the decisions of their Governing Bodies.

Article 2

2.1   WHO shall transmit relevant resolutions of the World Health Assembly and the recommendations of relevant WHO consultations, workshops and other official WHO meetings to OIE for the purpose of circulating them to OIE Members.

2.2   The OIE shall transmit the recommendations and resolutions of its International Committee as well as the recommendations of relevant OIE consultations, workshops and other official OIE meetings to WHO for the purpose of circulating them to WHO Member States.

2.3   These resolutions and recommendations sent for the consideration of the respective bodies of the two Organizations (hereinafter referred to as the Parties) shall form the basis for coordinated international action between the two Parties.

---

[1] Approved by the Fifty-seventh World Health Assembly on 22 May 2004 in resolution WHA57.7.

Article 3

3.1   Representatives of WHO shall be invited to attend the meetings of the International Committee and Regional Conferences of OIE and to participate without vote in the deliberations of these bodies with respect to items on their agenda in which WHO has an interest.

3.2   Representatives of OIE shall be invited to attend the meetings of the Executive Board and of the World Health Assembly and Regional Committees of WHO and to participate without vote in the deliberations of these bodies with respect to items on their agenda in which OIE has an interest.

3.3   Appropriate arrangements shall be made by agreement between the Director-General of WHO and the Director-General of OIE for participation of WHO and OIE in other meetings of a non-private character convened under their respective auspices which consider matters in which the other party has an interest; this especially involves those meetings leading to the definition of norms and standards.

3.4   The two Parties agree to avoid holding meetings and conferences dealing with matters of mutual interest without prior consultation with the other party.

Article 4

WHO and OIE shall collaborate in areas of common interest particularly by the following means:

4.1. Reciprocal exchange of reports, publications and other information, particularly the timely exchange of information on zoonotic and food-borne disease outbreaks. Special arrangements will be concluded between the two Parties to coordinate the response to outbreaks of zoonotic or/and foodborne diseases of recognized or potential international public health importance.

4.2   Organizing on both a regional and a world-wide basis meetings and conferences on zoonoses, food-borne diseases and related issues such as animal feeding practices and anti-microbial resistance related to the prudent use of anti-microbials in animal husbandry and their containment/control policies and programmes.

4.3   Joint elaboration, advocacy and technical support to national, regional or global programmes for the control or elimination of major zoonotic and food-borne diseases or emerging/ re-emerging issues of common interest.

4.4   Promoting and strengthening, especially in developing countries, VPH education, operationalization of VPH and effective co-operation between the public health and animal health/veterinary sectors.

4.5   International promotion and coordination of research activities on zoonoses, VPH and food safety.

4.6   Promoting and strengthening collaboration between the network of OIE Reference Centres and Laboratories and that of WHO Collaborating Centres and Reference Laboratories to consolidate their support to WHO Member States and OIE Members on issues of common interest.

Article 5

5.1   WHO and OIE will, in the course of the preparation of their respective programmes of work, exchange their draft programmes for comment.

5.2   Each party will take into account the recommendations of the other in preparing its final programme for submission to its governing body.

5.3   WHO and OIE will conduct one annual coordinating meeting of high level officials from headquarters and/or regional representation.

5.4   The two Parties should devise administrative arrangements necessary to implement these policies, such as the sharing of experts, common organization of joint scientific and technical meetings, joint training of health and veterinary personnel.

Article 6

6.1   The present Agreement shall enter into force on the date on which it is signed by the Director-General of WHO and the Director-General of the OIE, subject to the approval of the International Committee of the OIE and the World Health Assembly.

6.2   This Agreement may be modified by mutual consent expressed in writing. It may also be terminated by either party by giving 6 months' notice in writing to the other party.

Article 7

7.1   This Agreement supersedes the Agreement between the WHO and
      OIE adopted by WHO on 4 August 1960 and by the OIE on 8 August
      1960.

Signed in Geneva on 16 December 2004

for WHO   for OIE

LEE Jong-wook   Dr Bernard Vallat
Director-General   Director General

———————

PRINCIPLES GOVERNING RELATIONS BETWEEN THE WORLD HEALTH ORGANIZATION AND NONGOVERNMENTAL ORGANIZATIONS[1]

1. *Introduction*

1.1 As stated in Article 2 of the Constitution, one of the main functions of the World Health Organization (WHO) is to act as the directing and coordinating authority on international health work. In support of this function, and in accordance with Article 71 of the Constitution, WHO may make suitable arrangements for consultation and cooperation with nongovernmental organizations (NGOs) in carrying out its international health work.

1.2 WHO should, in relation to NGOs, act in conformity with any relevant resolutions of the General Assembly or Economic and Social Council of the United Nations.

1.3 The objectives of WHO's collaboration with NGOs are to promote the policies, strategies and programmes derived from the decisions of the Organization's governing bodies; to collaborate with regard to various WHO programmes in jointly agreed activities to implement these strategies; and to play an appropriate role in ensuring the harmonizing of intersectoral interests among the various sectoral bodies concerned in a country, regional or global setting.

2. *Types of relations at the global level and their development*

2.1 WHO recognizes only one category of *formal relations, known as official relations*, with those NGOs which meet the criteria described in these Principles. All other contacts, including working relations, are considered to be of an informal character.

2.2 The establishment of relations with NGOs shall be an evolving process proceeding through a number of separate stages as described in the following paragraphs.

2.3 First contacts with an NGO in order to create mutual understanding and assist in developing mutual interests frequently take the form of exchanges of information and reciprocal participation in technical meetings. This type of *informal contact* may continue on an *ad hoc* basis, without time limit

[1] Text adopted by the Fortieth World Health Assembly (resolution WHA40.25), in replacement of the Principles adopted by the First and Third World Health Assemblies.

and without written agreement. However, the definition of the broad objectives of collaboration and the possibility of enlarging its scope to include specific joint activities in line with the particular expertise of the nongovernmental organization are also explored at this stage.

2.4 When a number of specific joint activities have been identified, collaboration may be taken a stage further by proceeding to a period (usually two years) of *working relations* entered into by an exchange of letters. Such letters set out the agreed basis for the collaboration, indicating details of the activities to be undertaken during the period, providing an estimate of the resources to be supplied by WHO and the NGO, and naming focal points in the NGO and in WHO (designated technical officer). A joint assessment of the outcome of the collaboration thus planned is undertaken at the end of the period of working relations by the parties concerned, including also consideration of the future relationship. This may result: in the continuation of the working relations for a further period; in an application for admission into official relations with WHO from an international NGO, for examination by the Executive Board, should there be a number of activities which might form the basis of a long-term and closer relationship with WHO; or in a decision that there is no scope for further contacts in the foreseeable future. This arrangement for consultation and cooperation with NGOs is considered as informal.

2.5 The Executive Board shall be responsible for deciding on the admission of NGOs into *official relations* with WHO.

3. *Criteria for the admission of NGOs into official relations with WHO*

3.1 The main area of competence of the NGO shall fall within the purview of WHO. Its aims and activities shall be in conformity with the spirit, purposes and principles of the Constitution of WHO, shall centre on development work in health or health-related fields, and shall be free from concerns which are primarily of a commercial or profit-making nature. The major part of its activities shall be relevant to and have a bearing on the implementation of the health-for-all strategies as envisaged in the Global Strategy for Health for All by the Year 2000 and the WHO general programme of work covering a specific period.

3.2 The NGO shall normally be international in its structure and/or scope, and shall represent a substantial proportion of the persons globally organized for the purpose of participating in the particular field of interest in which it operates. When there are several international NGOs with similar areas of interest, they may form a joint committee or other body authorized to act for the group as a whole.

3.3 The NGO shall have a constitution or similar basic document, an established headquarters, a directing or governing body, an administrative structure at various levels of action, and authority to speak for its members through its authorized representatives. Its members shall exercise voting rights in relation to its policies or action.

3.4 Thus, organizations eligible for admission into official relations with WHO include various types of international NGOs with a federated structure (made up of national or regional groups or having individual members from different countries), foundations that raise resources for health development activities in different parts of the world, and similar bodies promoting international health.

3.5 In exceptional cases a national organization, whether or not affiliated to an international NGO, may be considered for admission into official relations, in consultation with and subject to the recommendations of the WHO Regional Director and the Member State involved. Such a national organization (or a number of national organizations working under a federated (umbrella) structure) shall be eligible for admission provided that: the major part of its activities and resources are directed towards international health and related work; it has developed a programme of collaborative activities with WHO as indicated in paragraph 2.4; and its activities offer appropriate experience upon which WHO may wish to draw.

3.6 There shall normally have been at least two years of successfully completed working relations, as described in paragraph 2.4, prior to an application for admission into official relations.

4. Procedure for admitting NGOs into official relations with WHO

4.1 Applications should normally reach WHO headquarters not later than the end of the month of July in order to be considered by the Executive Board in January of the following year. They shall specify a structured plan for collaborative activities agreed upon by the organization and WHO. Applications from national organizations shall contain the endorsements of the WHO Regional Director and the Government of the Member State concerned. Applications should normally be transmitted to Board members by the Secretariat two months in advance of the session at which they will be considered.

4.2 During its January session the Board's Standing Committee on Non-governmental Organizations, composed of five members, shall consider applications submitted by NGOs, voluntarily or by invitation, and shall make recommendations to the Board; it may invite any such organization to speak before it in connection with the organization's application. Should the applicant organization be considered not to meet the established criteria, and bearing in mind the desirability of ensuring a valuable continuing partnership based on defined objectives and evidenced by a record of successful past collaboration and a framework for future collaborative activities, the Standing Committee may recommend postponement of consideration or rejection of an application.

4.3 The Board, after considering the recommendations of the Standing Committee, shall decide whether an organization is to be admitted into official relations with WHO. A re-application from an NGO shall not normally be considered until two years have elapsed since the Board's decision on the original application.

4.4 The Director-General shall inform each organization of the Board's decision on its application. He shall maintain a list of the organizations admitted into official relations, and this list and any amendments thereto shall be circulated to the Members of WHO.

4.5 A plan for collaboration based on mutually agreed objectives and outlining activities for the coming three-year period shall form the basis of official relations between WHO and the NGO. This plan shall be transmitted also to the WHO regional offices to encourage closer collaboration at regional level as appropriate.

4.6 The Board, through its Standing Committee on Nongovernmental Organizations, shall review collaboration with each NGO every three years and shall determine the desirability of maintaining official relations. The Board's review shall be spread over a three-year period, one-third of the NGOs in official relations being reviewed each year.

4.7 The Board may discontinue official relations if it considers that such relations are no longer appropriate or necessary in the light of changing programmes or other circumstances. Similarly, the Board may suspend or discontinue official relations if an organization no longer meets the criteria that applied at the time of the establishment of such relations, or fails to fulfil its part in the agreed programme of collaboration.

5. Relations with NGOs at the regional and national levels[1]

5.1 Regional or national NGOs affiliated to international NGOs in official relations with WHO

These NGOs are, by definition, in official relations with the WHO regional office(s). They shall develop and implement a programme of collaboration with the regional and national levels of WHO to ensure implementation of health-for-all strategies at the country level.

5.2 Regional and national NGOs for which there is no international NGO

The regional office concerned may establish *working relations* with these organizations, subject to consultation between the Regional Director and the Director-General of WHO. A programme of activities developed and implemented as described in paragraph 2.4 would be essential.

5.3 Regional or national NGOs affiliated to international NGOs not in official relations with WHO

In order that WHO may promote and support the formation of strong international NGOs in the various technical fields, the regional office concerned may establish *working relations* with the above-mentioned regional or national organizations, subject to consultation between the Regional Director and the Director-General of WHO. Such working relations shall be based on a programme of activities developed and implemented as described in paragraph 2.4.

6. Privileges conferred on NGOs by relationship with WHO

6.1 The privileges conferred by official relationship shall include:

(i) the right to appoint a representative to participate, without right of vote, in WHO's meetings or in those of the committees and conferences convened under its authority, on the following conditions:

whenever the Health Assembly, or a committee or conference convened under WHO's authority, discusses an item in which a related NGO is particularly interested, that NGO, at the invitation of the chairman of the meeting or on his acceding to a request from the organization, shall be entitled to make a statement of an expository nature, and may, with the

---

[1] Before working relations are established between WHO and a national NGO, and before a programme of collaboration with such an organization is agreed, appropriate measures will be taken to consult the Government concerned in accordance with Article 71 of the WHO Constitution.

consent of the meeting, be invited by the chairman to make, in the course of the discussion of the item before the meeting, an additional statement for purposes of clarification;

(ii) access to non-confidential documentation and such other documentation as the Director-General may see fit to make available through such special distribution facilities as WHO may establish;

(iii) the right to submit a memorandum to the Director-General, who would determine the nature and scope of the circulation.

6.2 In the event of a memorandum being submitted which the Director-General considers might be placed on the agenda of the Health Assembly, such memorandum shall be placed before the Executive Board for possible inclusion in the agenda of the Assembly.

6.3 Privileges similar to those stated above shall normally be accorded to national/regional NGOs having working relations with WHO regional offices, in accordance with section 5, as determined by the Regional Directors in consultation with the regional committees.

6.4 A national organization which is affiliated to an international NGO covering the same subject on an international basis shall normally present its views through its government or through the international NGO to which it is affiliated, unless other arrangements are made in view of its particular relationship with WHO.

7. Responsibilities of NGOs in their relationship with WHO

7.1 NGOs shall be responsible for implementing the mutually agreed programme of collaboration and shall inform WHO as soon as possible if for any reason they are unable to fulfil their part of the agreement.

7.2 NGOs shall utilize the opportunities available to them through their normal work to disseminate information on WHO policies and programmes.

7.3 NGOs shall collaborate individually or collectively in WHO programmes to further health-for-all goals.

7.4 NGOs shall individually or collectively collaborate with the Member States where their activities are based in the implementation of the national/regional/global health-for-all strategies.

FINANCIAL REGULATIONS
OF THE WORLD HEALTH ORGANIZATION[1]

Regulation I – Applicability and Delegation of Authority

1.1 These Regulations shall govern the financial administration of the World Health Organization.

1.2 The Director-General is responsible for ensuring effective financial administration of the Organization in accordance with these Regulations.

1.3 Without prejudice to regulation 1.2 the Director-General may delegate in writing to other officers of the Organization such authority as he or she considers necessary for the effective implementation of these Regulations.

1.4 The Director-General shall establish Financial Rules, including relevant guidelines and limits for the implementation of these Regulations, in order to ensure effective financial administration, the exercise of economy, and safeguard of the assets of the Organization.

Regulation II – The Financial Period

2.1 The financial period shall be two consecutive calendar years beginning with an even-numbered year.

Regulation III – The Budget

3.1 The budget estimates for the financial period, as referred to in Article 55 of the Constitution (hereinafter referred to as "budget proposals"), shall be prepared by the Director-General.

3.2 The budget proposals shall cover gross income and gross expenditure for the financial period to which they relate, and shall be presented in United States dollars.

3.3 The budget proposals shall be divided into parts, sections and chapters, and shall include such information, annexes and explanatory statements as may be requested by, or on behalf of, the Health Assembly and such further annexes or statements as the Director-General may deem necessary and useful.

3.4 The Director-General shall submit the budget proposals at least twelve weeks before the opening of the regular session of the Health Assembly, and before the opening of the appropriate session of the Executive Board, at

[1] Text adopted by the Fifty-third World Health Assembly (resolution WHA53.6). Previous text adopted by the Fourth World Health Assembly (resolution WHA4.50) and amended by the Thirteenth, Eighteenth, Twenty-fifth, Twenty-sixth, Twenty-ninth, Thirtieth, Thirty-third, Thirty-seventh, Forty-first, Forty-fourth and Forty-eighth World Health Assemblies (resolutions WHA13.19, WHA18.13, WHA25.14, WHA25.15, WHA26.26, WHA29.27, WHA30.21, WHA33.8, WHA41.12, WHA44.16, WHA48.21 and decision WHA37(10)).

which they are to be considered. At the same time, the Director-General shall transmit these proposals to all Members (including Associate Members).

3.5 The Executive Board shall submit these proposals, and any recommendations it may have thereon, to the Health Assembly.

3.6 The budget for the following financial period shall be approved by the Health Assembly in the year preceding the biennium to which the budget proposals relate, after consideration and report on the proposals by the appropriate main committee of the Health Assembly.

3.7 Should the Director-General, at the time of the session of the Executive Board that submits the budget proposals and its recommendations thereon to the Health Assembly, have information which indicates that there may, before the time of the Health Assembly, be a need to alter the proposals in the light of developments, he or she shall report thereon to the Executive Board, which shall consider including in its recommendations to the Health Assembly an appropriate provision therefor.

3.8 Should developments subsequent to the session of the Executive Board that considers the budget proposals, or any of the recommendations made by it, necessitate or render desirable in the opinion of the Director-General an alteration in the budget proposals, the Director-General shall report thereon to the Health Assembly.

3.9 Supplementary proposals may be submitted to the Board by the Director-General whenever necessary to increase the appropriations previously approved by the Health Assembly. Such proposals shall be submitted in a form and manner consistent with the budget proposals for the financial period.

Regulation IV – Regular Budget Appropriations

4.1 The appropriations approved by the Health Assembly shall constitute an authorization to the Director-General to incur contractual obligations and make payments for the purposes for which the appropriations were approved and up to the amounts so approved.

4.2 Appropriations shall be available for obligation for the financial period to which they relate. The Director-General is authorized to charge, as an obligation against the appropriations during the current financial period, the cost of goods or services which were contracted during the current financial period, and which are to be supplied or rendered during that period or within the year following the end of the period.

4.3 The Director-General is authorized, with the prior concurrence of the Executive Board or of any committee to which it may delegate appropriate authority, to transfer credits between sections. When the Executive Board or any committee to which it may have delegated appropriate authority is not in session, the Director-General is authorized, with the prior written concurrence of the majority of the members of the Board or such committee, to transfer credits between sections. The Director-General shall report such transfers to the Executive Board at its next session.

4.4 At the same time as budget proposals are approved an exchange rate facility shall be established by the Health Assembly, which shall set the maximum level that may be available to cover losses on foreign exchange. The purpose of the facility shall be to make it possible to maintain the level of the budget so that the activities that are represented by the budget approved by the Health Assembly may be carried out irrespective of the effect of any fluctuation of currencies against the United States dollar at the official United Nations exchange rate. Any net gains or losses arising during the biennium shall be credited or debited to Miscellaneous Income.

4.5 Appropriations in respect of the regular budget for the current financial period may remain available for the following financial period to make it possible to carry forward unliquidated obligations in order to:

(*a*) complete activities for which the obligation was originally raised, provided that the implementation of these activities has commenced during the current financial period, by the end of the first year of the following financial period;

(*b*) pay for all goods and services rendered, under the unliquidated obligations referred to in regulation 4.5(*a*), by the end of the second year following that financial period.

4.6 At the end of the financial period, any unobligated balance of the appropriations shall be credited to Miscellaneous Income.

4.7 At the end of the financial period, any unliquidated obligations from the prior financial period shall be cancelled and credited to Miscellaneous Income.

4.8 Any claims that continue to exist against the Organization under unliquidated obligations cancelled in accordance with regulation 4.7 shall be transferred to new obligations against appropriations established for the current financial period.

Regulation V – Provision of Regular Budget Funds

5.1 Appropriations shall be financed by assessed contributions from Members, according to the scale of assessments determined by the Health Assembly, and by Miscellaneous Income.

5.2 The amount to be financed by contributions from Members shall be calculated after adjusting the total amount appropriated by the Health Assembly to reflect that proportion of the regular budget to be financed by Miscellaneous Income.

5.3 In the event that the amount realized as Miscellaneous Income is greater than the amount approved by the Health Assembly under the regular budget proposals, any such surplus shall be credited to Miscellaneous Income for the following financial period, and shall be applied in accordance with the budget approved for that financial period.

5.4 In the event that the amount realized as Miscellaneous Income is less than the amount approved by the Health Assembly under the regular budget proposals, the Director-General shall review implementation plans for the regular budget in order to make any adjustments that may be necessary.

Regulation VI – Assessed Contributions

6.1 The assessed contributions of Members based on the scale of assessments shall be divided into two equal annual instalments. In the first year of the financial period, the Health Assembly may decide to amend the scale of assessments to be applied to the second year of the financial period.

6.2 After the Health Assembly has adopted the budget, the Director-General shall inform Members of their commitments in respect of contributions for the financial period and request them to pay the first and second instalments of their contributions.

6.3 If the Health Assembly decides to amend the scale of assessments, or to adjust the amount of the appropriations to be financed by contributions from Members for the second year of a biennium, the Director-General shall inform Members of their revised commitments and shall request Members to pay the revised second instalment of their contributions.

6.4 Instalments of contributions shall be due and payable as of 1 January of the year to which they relate.

6.5 There shall be a financial incentive scheme which shall reward Member States that pay in full within the grace period set out in the Financial Rules. This financial incentive shall be calculated as a discount equivalent to interest calculated at the London Inter-bank Bid Rate for the period from the date of payment to the end of the grace period.

6.6 As of 1 January of the following year, the unpaid balance of such contributions shall be considered to be one year in arrears.

6.7 Contributions shall be assessed in United States dollars, and shall be paid in either United States dollars, euros or Swiss francs, or such other currency or currencies as the Director-General shall determine.

6.8 The acceptance by the Director-General of any currency that is not fully convertible shall be subject to a specific, annual approval on a case-by-case basis by the Director-General. Such approvals will include any terms and conditions that the Director-General considers necessary to protect the World Health Organization.

6.9 Payments made by a Member and/or credits from Miscellaneous Income shall be credited to the Member's account and applied first against the oldest amount outstanding.

6.10 Payments in currencies other than United States dollars shall be credited to Members' accounts at the United Nations rate of exchange ruling on the date of receipt by the World Health Organization.

6.11 The Director-General shall submit to the regular session of the Health Assembly a report on the collection of contributions.

6.12 New Members shall be required to make a contribution for the financial period in which they become Members at rates to be determined by the Health Assembly. When received, such unbudgeted assessments shall be credited to Miscellaneous Income.

Regulation VII – Working Capital Fund and Internal Borrowing

7.1 Pending the receipt of assessed contributions, implementation of the regular budget may be financed from the Working Capital Fund, which shall be established as part of the regular budget approved by the Health Assembly, and thereafter by internal borrowing against available cash reserves of the Organization, excluding Trust Funds.

7.2 The level of the Working Capital Fund shall be based on a projection of financing requirements taking into consideration projected income and expenditure. Any proposals that the Director-General may make to the Health Assembly for varying the level of the Working Capital Fund from that previously approved shall be accompanied by an explanation demonstrating the need for the change.

7.3 Any repayments of borrowing under regulation 7.1 shall be made from the collection of arrears of assessed contributions and shall be credited first against any internal borrowing outstanding and secondly against any borrowing outstanding from the Working Capital Fund.

Regulation VIII – Miscellaneous and other Income

8.1 Miscellaneous Income shall be applied in accordance with Regulation V and shall include the following:

(*a*) any unobligated balances within appropriations in accordance with regulation 4.6;

(*b*) any unliquidated obligations in accordance with regulation 4.7;

(c) any interest earnings or investment income on surplus liquidity in the regular budget;

(d) any refunds or rebates of expenditure received after the end of the financial period to which the original expenditure related;

(e) any proceeds of insurance claims that are not required to replace the insured item, or otherwise compensate for the loss;

(f) the net proceeds generated on the sale of a capital asset after allowing for all costs of acquisition, or improvement, of any asset concerned;

(g) any net gains or losses that may have arisen under operation of the exchange rate facility, or application of the official United Nations rates of exchange, or in revaluation for accounting purposes of the Organization's assets and liabilities;

(h) any payments of arrears of contributions due from Member States that are not required to repay borrowings from the Working Capital Fund or internal borrowing in accordance with regulation 7.3;

(i) any income not otherwise specifically referred to in these Regulations.

8.2 Any credits due to Members in accordance with regulation 6.5 shall be applied to offset Members' assessed contributions and shall be funded from Miscellaneous Income.

8.3 The Director-General is authorized to levy a charge on extrabudgetary contributions in accordance with any applicable resolution of the Health Assembly. This charge shall be used, together with any interest earnings or earnings from investments of extrabudgetary contributions, in accordance with regulation 11.3(b), to reimburse all, or part of, the indirect costs incurred by the Organization in respect of the generation and administration of extrabudgetary resources. All direct costs of the implementation of programmes that are financed by extrabudgetary resources shall be charged against the relevant extrabudgetary contribution.

8.4 Any refund of expenditure, or reimbursement for services and facilities provided, received from third parties during the biennium in which the original expenditure was incurred or services and facilities were provided shall be credited against that expenditure.

8.5 Any payments received from insurance policies held by the Organization shall be credited towards mitigating the loss that the insurance covered.

8.6 The Director-General is delegated the authority, under Article 57 of the Constitution, to accept gifts and bequests, either in cash or in kind, provided that he or she has determined that such contributions can be used by the Organization, and that any conditions which may be attached to them are consistent with the objective and policies of the Organization.

Regulation IX – Funds

9.1 Funds shall be established to enable the Organization to record income and expenditure. These funds shall cover all sources of income: regular budget, extrabudgetary resources, Trust Funds, and any other source of income as may be appropriate.

9.2 Accounts shall be established for amounts received from donors of extrabudgetary contributions and for any Trust Funds so that relevant income and expenditures may be recorded and reported upon.

9.3 Other accounts shall be established as necessary as reserves or to meet the requirements of the administration of the Organization, including capital expenditure.

9.4 The Director-General may establish revolving funds so that activities may be operated on a self-financing basis. The purpose of such accounts shall be reported to the Health Assembly, including details of sources of income and expenditures charged against such funds, and the disposition of any surplus balance at the end of a financial period.

9.5 The purpose of any account established under regulations 9.3 and 9.4 shall be specified and shall be subject to these Financial Regulations and such Financial Rules as are established by the Director-General under regulation 12.1, prudent financial management, and any specific conditions agreed with the appropriate authority.

Regulation X – Custody of Funds

10.1 The Director-General shall designate the bank or banks or financial institutions in which funds in the custody of the Organization shall be kept.

10.2 The Director-General may designate any investment (or asset) managers and/or custodians that the Organization may wish to appoint for the management of the funds in its custody.

Regulation XI – Investment of Funds

11.1 Any funds not required for immediate payment may be invested and may be pooled in so far as this benefits the return that may be generated.

11.2 Income from investments shall be credited to the fund or account from which invested moneys derive unless otherwise provided in the regulations, rules or resolutions relating to that fund or account.

11.3 (a) Income generated from regular budget resources shall be credited to Miscellaneous Income in accordance with regulation 8.1(c).

(b) Income generated from extrabudgetary resources may be used to reimburse indirect costs related to extrabudgetary resources.

11.4 Investment policies and guidelines shall be drawn up in accordance with best industry practice, having due regard for the preservation of capital and the return requirements of the Organization.

Regulation XII – Internal Control

12.1 The Director-General shall:

(*a*) establish operating policies and procedures in order to ensure effective financial administration, the exercise of economy, and safeguard of the assets of the Organization;

(*b*) designate the officers who may receive funds, incur financial commitments and make payments on behalf of the Organization;

(*c*) maintain an effective internal control structure to ensure the accomplishment of established objectives and goals for operations; the economical and efficient use of resources; the reliability and integrity of information; compliance with policies, plans, procedures, rules and regulations; and the safeguarding of assets;

(*d*) maintain an internal audit function which is responsible for the review, evaluation and monitoring of the adequacy and effectiveness of the Organization's overall systems of internal control. For this purpose, all systems, processes, operations, functions and activities within the Organization shall be subject to such review, evaluation and monitoring.

Regulation XIII – Accounts and Financial Reports

13.1 The Director-General shall establish such accounts as are necessary and shall, in so far as is not otherwise provided for in these Regulations and any Financial Rules established by the Director-General, maintain them in a manner consistent with the United Nations System Accounting Standards.

13.2 Final financial reports shall be prepared for each financial period, and interim financial reports shall be prepared at the end of the first year of each such period. Such financial reports shall be presented in conformity with – and in the formats established under – the Standards referred to in regulation 13.1, together with such other information as may be necessary to indicate the current financial position of the Organization.

13.3 The financial reports shall be presented in United States dollars. The accounting records may, however, be kept in such currency or currencies as the Director-General may deem necessary.

13.4 The financial reports shall be submitted to the External Auditor(s) not later than 31 March following the end of the financial period to which they relate.

13.5 The Director-General may make such ex gratia payments as deemed to be necessary in the interest of the Organization. A statement of such payments shall be included with the final accounts.

13.6 The Director-General may authorize, after full investigation, the writing-off of the loss of any asset, other than arrears of contributions. A statement of such losses written off shall be included with the final accounts.

Regulation XIV – External Audit

14.1 External Auditor(s), each of whom shall be the Auditor-General (or officer holding equivalent title or status) of a Member government, shall be appointed by the Health Assembly, in the manner decided by the Assembly. External Auditor(s) appointed may be removed only by the Assembly.

14.2 Subject to any special direction of the Health Assembly, each audit which the External Auditor(s) performs/perform shall be conducted in conformity with generally accepted common auditing standards and in accordance with the Additional Terms of Reference set out in the Appendix to these Regulations.

14.3 The External Auditor(s) may make observations with respect to the efficiency of the financial procedures, the accounting system, the internal financial controls and, in general, the administration and management of the Organization.

14.4 The External Auditor(s) shall be completely independent and solely responsible for the conduct of the audit.

14.5 The Health Assembly may request the External Auditor(s) to perform certain specific examinations and issue separate reports on the results.

14.6 The Director-General shall provide the External Auditor(s) with the facilities required for the performance of the audit.

14.7 For the purpose of making a local or special examination or for effecting economies of audit cost, the External Auditor(s) may engage the services of any national Auditor-General (or equivalent title) or commercial public auditors of known repute or any other person or firm that, in the opinion of the External Auditor(s), is technically qualified.

14.8 The External Auditor(s) shall issue a report on the audit of the biennium financial report prepared by the Director-General pursuant to Regulation XIII. The report shall include such information as he/she/they deem(s) necessary in regard to regulation 14.3 and the Additional Terms of Reference.

14.9 The report(s) of the External Auditor(s) shall be transmitted through the Executive Board, together with the audited financial report, to the

Health Assembly not later than 1 May following the end of the financial period to which the final accounts relate. The Executive Board shall examine the interim and biennium financial reports and the audit report(s) and shall forward them to the Health Assembly with such comments as it deems necessary.

Regulation XV – Resolutions involving Expenditures

15.1 Neither the Health Assembly nor the Executive Board shall take a decision involving expenditures unless it has before it a report from the Director-General on the administrative and financial implications of the proposal.

15.2 Where, in the opinion of the Director-General, the proposed expenditure cannot be made from the existing appropriations, it shall not be incurred until the Health Assembly has made the necessary appropriations.

Regulation XVI – General Provisions

16.1 These Regulations shall be effective as of the date of their approval by the Health Assembly, unless otherwise specified by the Health Assembly. They may be amended only by the Health Assembly.

16.2 In case of doubt as to the interpretation and application of any of the foregoing regulations, the Director-General is authorized to rule thereon, subject to confirmation by the Executive Board at its next session.

16.3 The Financial Rules established by the Director-General as referred to in regulation 1.4 above, and the amendments made by the Director-General to such rules, shall enter into force after confirmation by the Executive Board. They shall be reported upon to the Health Assembly for its information.

Appendix

ADDITIONAL TERMS
OF REFERENCE GOVERNING THE EXTERNAL AUDIT
OF THE WORLD HEALTH ORGANIZATION

1. The External Auditor(s) shall perform such audit of the accounts of the World Health Organization, including all Trust Funds and special accounts, as deemed necessary in order to satisfy himself/herself/themselves:

(*a*) that the financial statements are in accord with the books and records of the Organization;
(*b*) that the financial transactions reflected in the statements have been in accordance with the rules and regulations, the budgetary provisions, and other applicable directives;
(*c*) that the securities and moneys on deposit and on hand have been verified by the certificates received direct from the Organization's depositaries or by actual count;
(*d*) that the internal controls, including the internal audit, are adequate in the light of the extent of reliance placed thereon;
(*e*) that procedures satisfactory to the External Auditor(s) have been applied to the recording of all assets, liabilities, surpluses and deficits.

2. The External Auditor(s) shall be the sole judge as to the acceptance in whole or in part of certifications and representations by the Secretariat and may proceed to such detailed examination and verification as he/she/they choose(s) of all financial records including those relating to supplies and equipment.

3. The External Auditor(s) and staff shall have free access at all convenient times to all books, records and other documentation which are, in the opinion of the External Auditor(s), necessary for the performance of the audit. Information classified as privileged and which the Secretariat agrees is required by the External Auditor(s) for the purposes of the audit, and information classified as confidential, shall be made available on application. The External Auditor(s) and staff shall respect the privileged and confidential nature of any information so classified which has been made available and shall not make use of it except in direct connection with the performance of the audit. The External Auditor(s) may draw the attention of the Health Assembly to any denial of information classified as privileged which, in his/her/their opinion, was required for the purpose of the audit.

4. The External Auditor(s) shall have no power to disallow items in the accounts but shall draw to the attention of the Director-General for appropriate action any transaction that creates doubt as to legality or propriety. Audit objections, to these or any other transactions, arising during the examination of the accounts shall be immediately communicated to the Director-General.

5. The External Auditor(s) shall express and sign an opinion on the financial statements of the Organization. The opinion shall include the following basic elements:

(*a*) identification of the financial statements audited;
(*b*) a reference to the responsibility of the entity's management and responsibility of the External Auditor(s);
(*c*) a reference to the audit standards followed;
(*d*) a description of the work performed;
(*e*) an expression of opinion on the financial statements as to whether:
(i) the financial statements present fairly the financial position as at the end of the period and the results of the operations for the period;
(ii) the financial statements were prepared in accordance with the stated accounting policies;
(iii) the accounting policies were applied on a basis consistent with that of the preceding financial period;
(*f*) an expression of opinion on the compliance of transactions with the Financial Regulations and legislative authority;
(*g*) the date of the opinion;
(*h*) the External Auditor's(s') name and position;
(*i*) the place where the report has been signed;
(*j*) should it be necessary, a reference to the report of the External Auditor(s) on the financial statements.

6. The report of the External Auditor(s) to the Health Assembly on the financial operations of the period should mention:

(*a*) the type and scope of examination;

(*b*) matters affecting the completeness or accuracy of the accounts, including where appropriate:

(i) information necessary to the correct interpretation of the accounts;

(ii) any amounts that ought to have been received but which have not been brought to account;

(iii) any amounts for which a legal or contingent obligation exists and which have not been recorded or reflected in the financial statements;

(iv) expenditures not properly substantiated;

(v) whether proper books of accounts have been kept; where in the presentation of statements there are deviations of a material nature from a consistent application of generally accepted accounting principles, these should be disclosed;

(*c*) other matters that should be brought to the notice of the Health Assembly such as:

(i) cases of fraud or presumptive fraud;

(ii) wasteful or improper expenditure of the Organization's money or other assets (notwithstanding that the accounting for the transaction may be correct);

(iii) expenditure likely to commit the Organization to further outlay on a large scale;

(iv) any defect in the general system or detailed regulations governing the control of receipts and disbursements, or of supplies and equipment;

(v) expenditure not in accordance with the intention of the Health Assembly, after making allowance for duly authorized transfers within the budget;

(vi) expenditure in excess of appropriations as amended by duly authorized transfers within the budget;

(vii) expenditure not in conformity with the authority that governs it;

(*d*) the accuracy or otherwise of the supplies and equipment records as determined by stock-taking and examination of the records.

In addition, the report may contain reference to:

(*e*) transactions accounted for in a previous financial period, concerning which further information has been obtained, or transactions in a later financial period concerning which it seems desirable that the Health Assembly should have early knowledge.

7. The External Auditor(s) may make such observations with respect to his/her/their findings resulting from the audit and such comments on the financial report as he/she/they deem(s) appropriate to the Health Assembly or to the Director-General.

8. Whenever the External Auditor's(s') scope of audit is restricted, or insufficient evidence is available, the External Auditor's(s') opinion shall refer to this matter, making clear in the report the reasons for the comments and the effect on the financial position and the financial transactions as recorded.

9. In no case shall the External Auditor(s) include criticism in any report without first affording the Director-General an adequate opportunity of explanation on the matter under observation.

10. The External Auditor(s) is/are not required to mention any matter referred to in the foregoing which is considered immaterial.

STAFF REGULATIONS OF THE WORLD HEALTH ORGANIZATION[1]

SCOPE AND PURPOSE

The Staff Regulations embody the fundamental conditions of service and the basic rights, duties and obligations of the World Health Organization Secretariat staff. They are the broad principles of personnel policy for the guidance of the Director-General in the staffing and administration of the Secretariat. The Director-General may, as Chief Administrative Officer, provide and enforce such Staff Rules consistent with these principles as he considers necessary.

I. DUTIES, OBLIGATIONS AND PRIVILEGES

1.1 All staff members of the Organization are international civil servants. Their responsibilities are not national but exclusively international. By accepting appointment, they pledge themselves to discharge their functions and to regulate their conduct with the interests of the World Health Organization only in view.

1.2 All staff members are subject to the authority of the Director-General and to assignment by him to any of the activities or offices of the World Health Organization. They are responsible to him in the exercise of their functions. In principle, the whole time of staff members shall be at the disposal of the Director-General.

1.3 In the performance of their duties staff members shall neither seek nor accept instructions from any government or from any other authority external to the Organization.

1.4 No staff member shall accept, hold or engage in any office or occupation which is incompatible with the proper discharge of his duties with the World Health Organization.

1.5 Staff members shall conduct themselves at all times in a manner compatible with their status as international civil servants. They shall avoid any action and in particular any kind of public pronouncement which may adversely reflect on their status. While they are not expected to give up their national sentiments or their political and religious convictions, they

[1] Text adopted by the Fourth World Health Assembly (resolution WHA4.51) and amended by the Twelfth and Fifty-fifth World Health Assemblies (Resolutions WHA12.33 and WHA55.21).

Staff Regulations

shall at all times bear in mind the reserve and tact incumbent upon them by reason of their international status.

1.6 Staff members shall exercise the utmost discretion in regard to all matters of official business. They shall not communicate to any person any information known to them by reason of their official position which has not been made public, except in the course of their duties or by authorization of the Director-General. At no time shall they in any way use to private advantage information known to them by reason of their official position. These obligations do not cease with separation from service.

1.7 No staff member shall accept any honour, decoration, favour, gift or remuneration from any government, or from any other source external to the Organization, if such acceptance is incompatible with his status as an international civil servant.

1.8 Any staff member who becomes a candidate for a public office of a political character shall resign from the Secretariat.

1.9 The immunities and privileges attaching to the World Health Organization by virtue of Article 67 of the Constitution are conferred in the interests of the Organization. These privileges and immunities furnish no excuse to staff members for non-performance of their private obligations or failure to observe laws and police regulations. The decision whether to waive any privileges or immunities of the staff in any case that arises shall rest with the Director-General.

1.10 All staff members shall subscribe to the following oath or declaration: I solemnly swear (undertake, affirm, promise) to exercise in all loyalty, discretion, and conscience the functions entrusted to me as an international civil servant of the World Health Organization, to discharge those functions and regulate my conduct with the interests of the World Health Organization only in view, and not to seek or accept instructions in regard to the performance of my duties from any government or other authority external to the Organization.

1.11 The oath or declaration shall be made orally by the Director-General at a public meeting of the World Health Assembly, by the Deputy Director-General, Assistant Directors-General and Regional Directors before the Director-General and in writing by other staff members.

II. CLASSIFICATION OF POSTS AND STAFF

2.1 Appropriate provision shall be made by the Director-General for the classification of posts and staff according to the nature of the duties and responsibilities required.

III. Salaries and Related Allowances

3.1 The salaries for the Deputy Director-General, Assistant Directors-General and Regional Directors shall be determined by the World Health Assembly on the recommendation of the Director-General and with the advice of the Executive Board.

3.2 Salary levels for other staff shall be determined by the Director-General on the basis of their duties and responsibilities. The salary and allowance plan shall be determined by the Director-General following basically the scales of salaries and allowances of the United Nations, provided that for staff occupying positions subject to local recruitment the Director-General may establish salaries and allowances in accordance with best prevailing local practices and that for staff occupying positions subject to international recruitment the remuneration shall be varied between duty stations to take into account relative cost of living to the staff members concerned, standards of living and related factors. Any deviations from the United Nations scales of salaries and allowances which may be necessary for the requirements of the World Health Organization shall be subject to the approval of, or may be authorized by, the Executive Board.

IV. Appointment and Promotion

4.1 The Director-General shall appoint staff members as required.

4.2 The paramount consideration in the appointment, transfer or promotion of the staff shall be the necessity of securing the highest standards of efficiency, competence and integrity. Due regard shall be paid to the importance of recruiting and maintaining the staff on as wide a geographical basis as possible.

4.3 Selection of staff members shall be without regard to race, creed or sex. So far as is practicable, selection shall be made on a competitive basis.

4.4 Without prejudice to the inflow of fresh talent at the various levels, vacancies shall be filled by promotion of persons already in the service of the Organization in preference to persons from outside. This preference shall also be applied, on a reciprocal basis, to the United Nations and specialized agencies brought into relationship with the United Nations.

4.5 Appointments of the Deputy Director-General, Assistant Directors-General and Regional Directors shall be for a period not to exceed five years, subject to renewal, and in accordance with conditions determined by the Executive Board concerning eligibility of Regional Directors for reappointment. Other staff members shall be granted appointments of a duration and under such terms and conditions, consistent with these regulations, as the Director-General may prescribe.

4.6 The Director-General shall establish appropriate medical standards which prospective staff members shall normally be required to meet before appointment.

V. ANNUAL AND SPECIAL LEAVE

5.1 Staff members shall be allowed appropriate annual leave. In exceptional cases, special leave may be authorized by the Director-General.

5.2 In order that staff members may take their leave periodically in their home countries, the Organization shall allow necessary travelling time for that purpose, under conditions and definitions prescribed by the Director-General.

VI. SOCIAL SECURITY

6.1 Provision shall be made for the participation of staff members in the United Nations Joint Staff Pension Fund in accordance with the regulations of that fund.

6.2 The Director-General shall establish a scheme of social security for the staff, including provisions for health protection, sick leave and maternity leave, and reasonable compensation in the event of illness, accident or death attributable to the performance of official duties on behalf of the Organization.

VII. TRAVEL AND REMOVAL EXPENSES

7.1 Subject to conditions and definitions prescribed by the Director-General, the Organization shall pay the travel expenses of staff members and, in appropriate cases, their dependants

upon appointment and on subsequent change of official duty station,

upon the taking of leave at home when authorized, and

upon separation from the service.

7.2 Subject to conditions and definitions prescribed by the Director-General, the World Health Organization shall pay removal costs for staff members

upon appointment and on subsequent change of official duty station and

upon separation from the service.

VIII. STAFF RELATIONS

8.1 The Director-General shall make provision for staff participation in the discussion of policies relating to staff questions.

IX. SEPARATION FROM SERVICE

9.1 Staff members may resign from the Secretariat upon giving the Director-General the notice required under the terms of their appointment.

9.2 The Director-General may terminate the appointment of a staff member in accordance with the terms of his appointment, or if the necessities of the service require abolition of the post or reduction of the staff, if the services of the individual concerned prove unsatisfactory, or if he is, for reasons of health, incapacitated for further service.

9.3 If the Director-General terminates an appointment the staff member shall be given notice and indemnity payment in accordance with the terms of his appointment.

9.4 The Director-General shall establish a scheme for the payment of repatriation grants.

9.5 Normally, staff members shall not be retained in active service beyond the age specified in the Pension Fund regulations as the age of retirement. The Director-General may, in the interests of the Organization, extend this age limit in exceptional cases.

X. DISCIPLINARY MEASURES

10.1 The Director-General may impose disciplinary measures on staff members whose conduct is unsatisfactory. He may summarily dismiss a member of the staff for serious misconduct.

XI. APPEALS

11.1 The Director-General shall establish administrative machinery with staff participation to advise him in case of any appeal by staff members against an administrative decision alleging the non-observance of their terms of appointment, including all pertinent regulations and rules, or against disciplinary action.

11.2 Any dispute which cannot be resolved internally, arising between the Organization and a member of the staff regarding the fulfilment of the contract of the said member, shall be referred for final decision to the United Nations Administrative Tribunal.

XII. GENERAL PROVISIONS

12.1 These regulations may be supplemented or amended by the Health Assembly, without prejudice to the acquired rights of staff members.

12.2 The Director-General shall report annually to the Health Assembly such staff rules and amendments thereto as he may make to implement these regulations, after confirmation by the Executive Board.

12.3 The Director-General, by virtue of the authority vested in him as the chief technical and administrative officer of the Organization, may delegate to other officers of the Organization such of his powers as he considers necessary for the effective implementation of these regulations.

12.4 In case of doubt as to the meaning of any of the foregoing regulations, the Director-General is authorized to rule thereon subject to confirmation of the ruling by the Executive Board at its next meeting.

REGULATIONS FOR EXPERT ADVISORY PANELS AND COMMITTEES[1]

INTRODUCTION

Efficiency, as well as economy, makes it necessary to limit the number of experts participating in discussions on any given subject; on the other hand, it is difficult, in a small group of experts, to obtain adequate representation of the various branches of knowledge which bear upon its subject, and of the diversified forms of local experience and trends of thought prevailing in the various parts of the world.

These apparently conflicting requirements may be reconciled by giving expert committees, whenever desirable, flexible membership.

This may be done by setting up advisory panels of experts conversant with all the required branches of knowledge and forms of experience needed to cover adequately a particular subject and providing adequate geographical representation.

From these panels will be drawn the members of the expert committees, selection being made according to the agenda of each meeting.

The following regulations are, therefore, based on the above principles.

1. DEFINITIONS

1.1 An expert advisory panel consists of experts from whom the Organization may obtain technical guidance and support within a particular subject, either by correspondence or at meetings to which the experts may be invited.

1.2 A member of an expert advisory panel is an expert appointed by the Director-General who undertakes to contribute by correspondence technical information on developments in his or her field, and to offer advice as appropriate, spontaneously or upon request.

1.3 An expert committee is a group of expert advisory panel members convened by the Director-General for the purpose of reviewing and making technical recommendations on a subject of interest to the Organization.

---

[1] Text adopted by the Thirty-fifth World Health Assembly (resolution WHA35.10), in replacement of the regulations adopted by the Fourth World Health Assembly. Amendments were adopted at the Forty-fifth, Forty-ninth, Fifty-third and Fifty-fifth World Health Assemblies (decision WHA45(10), resolution WHA49.29, resolution WHA53.8 and resolution WHA55.24, respectively).

1.4 A member of an expert committee is an expert appointed by the Director-General to serve at any particular meeting of that committee.

2. AUTHORITY TO ESTABLISH
EXPERT ADVISORY PANELS AND COMMITTEES

2.1 An expert advisory panel may be established by the Director-General in any field as and when required by the development of the Organization's programme. It is established for the Organization as a whole and shall be utilized at whatever level of operation its guidance and support are needed. An expert advisory panel may be disestablished by the Director-General at his discretion when its guidance and support are no longer required.

2.2 The Director-General shall report to the Executive Board on the establishment or disestablishment of expert advisory panels and on their membership.

2.3 The World Health Assembly and the Executive Board have authority under Articles 18(e) and 38 of the Constitution of the Organization to establish and dissolve expert committees.

2.4 The Director-General shall include in his biennial programme budget such proposals for expert committee meetings as he deems necessary.

3. EXPERT ADVISORY PANELS –
MEMBERSHIP AND PROCEDURES

3.1 Any person possessing qualifications and/or experience relevant and useful to the activities of the Organization in a field covered by an established expert advisory panel may be considered for appointment as a member of that panel after consultations with the national authorities concerned. Information on all appointments made to these panels shall be circulated to all Member States. The Director-General shall encourage developing countries to send nominations for the panels.

3.2 In the selection of members of expert advisory panels the Director-General shall consider primarily their technical ability and experience, but he shall also endeavour to ensure that the panels have the broadest possible international representation in terms of diversity of knowledge, experience and approaches in the fields for which the panels are established. He/she shall encourage nomination of experts from developing countries and from all regions and shall be helped in this task by Regional Directors.

3.3 Members of expert advisory panels shall be appointed for such period as the Director-General may determine, but not exceeding four years.

3.3.1 At the expiration of that period, the appointment shall end. However, the Director-General may renew the appointment when such renewal is warranted by specific programme requirements. Renewals of appointments should be fixed for periods of up to four years.

3.3.2 The appointment shall also end if the panel is disestablished. It may also be terminated at any time by the Director-General if the interests of the Organization so require. The Director-General shall report to the Executive Board on any such early termination of appointment.

3.4 Members of expert advisory panels do not receive any remuneration from the Organization. However, when attending meetings by invitation of WHO, they shall be entitled, in accordance with the administrative regulations of the Organization, to reimbursement of travelling expenses and to a daily living allowance during such meetings.

4. EXPERT COMMITTEES – MEMBERSHIP AND PROCEDURES

Selection, Appointment and Term of Office of Members

4.1 The Director-General shall establish the number of experts to be invited to a meeting of an expert committee, determine its date and duration, and convene the committee.

4.2 As a general rule, the Director-General shall select from one or more expert advisory panels the members of an expert committee on the basis of the principles of equitable geographical representation, gender balance, a balance of experts from developed and developing countries, representation of different trends of thought, approaches and practical experience in various parts of the world, and an appropriate interdisciplinary balance. The membership of expert committees shall not be restricted by consideration of language, within the range of languages of the Organization.

4.3 Members of an expert advisory panel who are not invited to a particular meeting of an expert committee of interest to them may at their request attend as observers, if so authorized by the Director-General, but shall do so at their own expense.

4.4 Organizations of the United Nations system, as well as nongovernmental organizations in official relations with WHO, may be invited to send representatives to expert committee meetings in which they are directly interested.

4.5 To ensure balanced geographical representation, consultants and temporary advisers assigned to assist an expert committee shall be selected, as far as possible, from countries not represented on the committee's membership.

International Status of Members

4.6 In the exercise of their functions, the members of expert advisory panels and committees shall act as international experts serving the Organization exclusively; in that capacity they may not request or receive instructions from any government or authority external to the Organization. Furthermore, they shall disclose all circumstances that could give rise to a potential conflict of interest as a result of their membership of an expert committee, in accordance with the mechanisms established by the Director-General for that purpose.

4.7 They shall enjoy the privileges and immunities envisaged in Article 67(*b*) of the Constitution of the Organization and set forth in the Convention on the Privileges and Immunities of the Specialized Agencies and in Annex VII thereof.

Agenda

4.8 The Director-General, or his representative, shall prepare the draft agenda for each meeting and transmit it in reasonable time to the members of the committee and of the Executive Board, and to Members of the Organization. An expert committee, unless formally so requested, may not deal with questions of administrative policy. The agenda shall include any subject, within the terms of reference of the committee, proposed by the Health Assembly, the Executive Board or the Director-General.

4.9 In order to provide members of an expert committee with the broadest possible information on the subjects under discussion, the terms of reference and annotated agenda of the meeting shall be supplied in advance to members of expert advisory panels who are conversant with these subjects but have not been invited to the meeting. They may also be invited to provide written contributions and may receive the principal working documents.

Expert Sub-committees

4.10 For the study of special problems a committee may suggest the establishment, temporarily or permanently, of specialized sub-committees, and may make suggestions as to their composition. A committee may also suggest the establishment of joint sub-committees consisting of specialists in its own technical field and of specialists in another field whose collaboration it considers necessary for the success of its work. The Health Assembly, or the Executive Board, shall decide whether such sub-committees shall be established, and whether singly or jointly with other committees or sub-committees of the Organization.

4.11 The rules governing the functions of committees, the appointment of their members, the election of their chairmen and vice-chairmen, secretary-ship and agenda shall, *mutatis mutandis*, apply to sub-committees. Membership of a committee does not in itself entitle an expert to participate in the proceedings of any of its sub-committees.

Reports on Meetings of Committees

4.12 For each meeting an expert committee shall draw up a report setting forth its findings, observations and recommendations. This report shall be completed and approved by the expert committee before the end of its meeting. Its conclusions and recommendations shall not commit the Organization and should be formulated in such a way as to advise the Director-General on future programme activities without calling upon him to use the staff, services or funds of the Organization in any specified way. If the committee is not unanimous in its findings, any divergent views shall be recorded in or appended to the report. Signed contributions may not be included in the text of the expert committee's report or in its annexes.

4.13 The text of an expert committee report may not be modified without the committee's consent. The Director-General may direct to the attention of the chairman of an expert committee any statement of opinion in its report that might be considered prejudicial to the best interests of the Organization or of any Member State. The chairman of the committee may, at his discretion, delete such statement from the report, with or without communicating with members of the expert committee, or, after obtaining their written approval, may modify the statement. Any difficulty arising out of a divergence of views between the Director-General and the chairman of the committee shall be referred to the Executive Board.

4.14 The Director-General shall be responsible for authorizing the publication of reports of expert committees. Nevertheless, the Director-General may communicate the report directly to the Health Assembly if, in his opinion, it contains information or advice urgently required by that body.

4.15 The Director-General may publish or authorize the publication of any document prepared for an expert committee, with due recognition of authorship if applicable.

Reports on Meetings of Sub-committees

4.16 The above provisions (paragraphs 4.12-4.15) shall apply to reports on meetings of sub-committees, except that the report of a sub-committee or joint sub-committee shall be submitted through the Director-General to the parent committee or committees. Nevertheless, the Director-General may communicate the report of a sub-committee directly to the Executive Board or to the Health Assembly if, in his opinion, it contains information or advice urgently required by either of those bodies.

Venue of Meetings of Committees

4.17 Meetings of expert committees shall normally be held at headquarters in order to provide overall technical guidance. They may also be convened at regional level, to deal with problems of a predominantly regional character, or at country level, if the health problems under consideration are essentially country-specific. Meetings of such expert committees shall be planned in a coordinated manner so as to complement those convened at headquarters, avoid duplication, and ensure maximum effectiveness and coherence in their work.

4.18 The above provisions (paragraphs 4.1-4.15) shall be applicable, *mutatis mutandis*, to expert committees that meet at the regional or country level. The Director-General may delegate the necessary authority to the Regional Directors.

Rules of Procedure

4.19 Expert committees and sub-committees shall conduct their proceedings in accordance with the Rules of Procedure set forth in the annex to these regulations.

Joint Committees and Sub-committees

4.20 The selection and appointment of expert advisory panel members designated by the Director-General to serve on a joint committee or sub-committee convened by the Organization in conjunction with other organizations shall also be governed by these regulations. In this selection, account shall be taken of the technical and geographical balance that is desirable for the joint committee or sub-committee as a whole.

4.21 Members of expert advisory panels appointed by the Director-General to such joint committees and sub-committees shall retain complete freedom of opinion and expression. Therefore their participation in any collective decision which may entail administrative, financial or moral responsibility for another participating organization does not commit the Organization.

4.22 Members of expert advisory panels representing the Organization on any joint committee or sub-committee shall report to the Director-General on their participation. This report shall be supplementary to the collective report of the joint committee or sub-committee itself.

Reporting to the Executive Board

4.23 The Director-General shall submit to the Executive Board a report on meetings of expert committees held since the previous session of the Board. It shall contain his observations on the implications of the expert committee reports and his recommendations on the follow-up action to be taken, and the texts of the recommendations of the expert committee shall be annexed. The Executive Board shall consider the report submitted by the Director-General and address its comments to it.

5. ENTRY-INTO-FORCE

5.1 These regulations shall apply as from the date of their approval by the Health Assembly.

Annex

RULES OF PROCEDURE FOR EXPERT COMMITTEES

PRIVATE NATURE OF MEETINGS

Rule 1

The meetings of expert committees shall normally be of a private character. They cannot become public except by the express decision of the committee with the full agreement of the Director-General.

QUORUM

Rule 2

The discussions of an expert committee shall be valid:

(a) if at least two-thirds of its members are present; and

(b) if, unless otherwise authorized by the Director-General, a representative of the Director-General is also present.

CHAIRMAN, VICE-CHAIRMAN AND RAPPORTEUR

Rule 3

The expert committee shall elect, from among its members, a chairman to direct its debates, a vice-chairman to replace the chairman if necessary, and a rapporteur.

SECRETARYSHIP

Rule 4

1. In accordance with Article 32 of the Constitution of the Organization, the Director-General is *ex-officio* secretary of all expert committees. He may delegate those functions to a technical officer competent in the subject concerned.

2. The Director-General, or his representative, may at any time make either oral or written statements to the committee concerning any question under consideration.

3. The Director-General, or his representative, shall determine the time and place of the meeting and shall convene the committee.

4. The committee's secretariat, composed of the secretary and of staff members, consultants and temporary advisers, as required, shall assist the chairman, the rapporteur and the members of the committee.

AGENDA

Rule 5

1. The secretary of the meeting shall prepare the draft agenda, submit it to the Director-General for approval, and transmit it to the members of the committee together with the letter of invitation to the meeting.

2. The agenda shall include any subject within the terms of reference of the committee proposed by the Health Assembly, the Executive Board or the Director-General.

VOTE

Rule 6

Scientific questions shall not be submitted to a vote. If the members of a committee cannot agree, each shall be entitled to have his personal opinion reflected in the report; this statement of opinion shall take the form of an individual or group report, stating the reasons why a divergent opinion is held.

CONDUCT OF BUSINESS

Rule 7

Save as provided in Rule 6 above, the chairman shall be guided by the provisions of the Rules of Procedure of the Executive Board on the conduct of business and voting in the committee in so far as this may be necessary for the accomplishment of the work of the committee.

REPORTS

Rule 8

The expert committee shall draw up and approve its report before the closure of its meeting.

WORKING LANGUAGES

Rule 9

1. The working languages of the expert committee shall be English and French. The Secretariat shall make such arrangements as are necessary to provide for interpretation from and into the other official languages of the Health Assembly and the Executive Board.

2. For expert committees held at regional or country level, working languages of that region other than English and French may be chosen as the committee's working languages; arrangements may be made for interpretation from and into other languages as required.

REGULATIONS FOR STUDY AND SCIENTIFIC GROUPS, COLLABORATING INSTITUTIONS AND OTHER MECHANISMS OF COLLABORATION[1]

INTRODUCTION

The World Health Organization requires expert advice for overall scientific and technical guidance, as well as for direct support of global, interregional and regional technical cooperation programmes for national health development.

Such advice and support must reflect high scientific and technical standards, the widest possible representation of different branches of knowledge, and local experience and trends of thought throughout the world, and must cover a broad range of disciplines related to health and social development.

Expert advice and support may be obtained from and provided by individuals, groups and institutions.

The present regulations do not cover:

(*a*) advice obtained from members of expert advisory panels acting individually or collaborating in expert committees;[2]

(*b*) expert advice available informally;

(*c*) expertise provided at regional level on problems of a regional or subregional character;

(*d*) advice obtained through channels covered by other regulations (e.g. from non-governmental organizations); or

(*e*) scientific and technical meetings other than those of expert committees, study groups and scientific groups, and especially meetings concerned with and adapted to special programmes (e.g. the Special Programme for Research and Training in Tropical Diseases, the Special Programme of Research, Development and Research Training in Human Reproduction, the Diarrhoeal Diseases Control Programme, the International Programme on Chemical Safety).

Adherence to the principles underlying these regulations is essential, but practical application must be responsive to evolving demands on the Organization, and new ways and means of securing and using expertise may prove necessary.

---

[1] Text approved by the Executive Board at its sixty-ninth session (resolution EB69.R21) with amendments approved at its 105th session (resolution EB105.R7).
[2] For regulations for expert advisory panels and committees, see p. 105.

1. STUDY GROUPS

1.1 Study groups may be convened instead of expert committees when one or more of the following conditions are met:

- the knowledge on the subject to be studied is still too uncertain and the opinions of competent specialists are too diverse for there to be a reasonable expectation of authoritative conclusions which can be immediately utilized by the Organization;

- the study envisaged concerns too limited an aspect of a general problem, which may or may not come within the purview of an expert committee;

- the study envisaged implies the collaboration of narrowly specialized participants who may belong to very different disciplines and on whom the Organization occasionally calls, without its being necessary, however, to include them in its expert advisory panels;

- certain non-technical factors render unsuitable an expert committee meeting, which would be too official in character;

- urgent or exceptional circumstances call for some administrative procedure which will be simpler and more rapidly applicable than that involved in meetings of expert committees.

1.2 The Director-General has authority to convene study groups, to determine the nature and scope of their subjects, the date and duration of their meetings, their membership, and whether their reports should be published. In so doing, the Director-General shall follow, whenever applicable and as far as practicable, the principles and rules applicable to expert committees, particularly those concerning the technical and geographical balance of the groups. Members of study groups may be members of expert advisory panels or other experts.

1.3 The regulations applying to the reports and documents of expert committees shall also apply to the reports and documents of study groups.

1.4 Meetings of study groups may be held at the regional level, to deal with subjects essentially of regional interest, when one or more of the conditions outlined in paragraph 1.1 above are met. Such study groups may be convened by Regional Directors, who will apply to them the provisions of regulation 1.2 above, *mutatis mutandis*, and ensure optimal coordination between such study group meetings and meetings on the same or related subjects in other regions or at headquarters level.

1.5 Should a study group be convened in conjunction with another organization, regulations 4.20 to 4.22 concerning expert advisory panels and committees shall apply, *mutatis mutandis*.

1.6 In the exercise of their functions the members of WHO expert advisory panels and other experts participating in study group meetings shall act as international experts serving the Organization exclusively; in that capacity they may not request or receive instructions from any government or authority external to the Organization. They shall enjoy the privileges and immunities envisaged in Article 67(*b*) of the Constitution of the Organization and set forth in the Convention on the Privileges and Immunities of the Specialized Agencies and in Annex VII thereof.

2. SCIENTIFIC GROUPS

2.1 The functions of scientific groups are to review given fields of medical, health and health systems research, to assess the current state of knowledge in those fields, and to determine how that knowledge may best be extended. In other words, scientific groups play for research a role comparable to that of expert committees and study groups for the Organization's programme in general.

2.2 The Director-General has authority to convene scientific groups and to determine the nature and scope of their subjects, the date and duration of their meetings, and their membership. In so doing, the Director-General should follow, whenever applicable and as far as practicable, the principles and rules applicable to expert committees. Members of scientific groups may be members of expert advisory panels or other experts.

2.3 The Director-General shall submit the reports of scientific groups to the global Advisory Committee on Health Research,[1] and the reports may be published at his discretion.

2.4 Meetings of scientific groups may be held at the regional level, to deal with subjects essentially of regional interest. Such scientific groups may be convened by Regional Directors, who will apply to them the provisions of regulation 2.2 above, *mutatis mutandis*, and ensure optimal coordination between such scientific group meetings and meetings on the same or related subjects in other regions or at headquarters level.

2.5 Should a scientific group be convened in conjunction with another organization, regulations 4.20 to 4.22 concerning expert advisory panels and committees shall apply, *mutatis mutandis*.

---

[1] The former title (Advisory Committee on Medical Research) was changed by the Thirty-ninth World Health Assembly in its decision WHA39(8).

2.6 In the exercise of their functions the members of WHO expert advisory panels and other experts participating in scientific group meetings shall act as international experts serving the Organization exclusively; in that capacity they may not request or receive instructions from any government or authority external to the Organization. They shall enjoy the privileges and immunities envisaged in Article 67(*b*) of the Constitution of the Organization and set forth in the Convention on the Privileges and Immunities of the Specialized Agencies and in Annex VII thereof.

3. WHO COLLABORATING CENTRES

Definition and Functions

3.1 A WHO collaborating centre is an institution designated by the Director-General to form part of an international collaborative network carrying out activities in support of the Organization's programme at all levels. A department or laboratory within an institution or a group of facilities for reference, research or training belonging to different institutions may be designated as a centre, one institution acting for them in relations with the Organization.

3.2 Institutions showing a growing capacity to fulfil a function or functions related to the Organization's programme, as well as institutions of high scientific and technical standing having attained international recognition, may qualify for designation as WHO collaborating centres.

3.3 The functions of WHO collaborating centres, severally or collectively, include the following:

(*a*) collection, collation and dissemination of information;

(*b*) standardization of terminology and nomenclature, of technology, of diagnostic, therapeutic and prophylactic substances, and of methods and procedures;

(*c*) development and application of appropriate technology;

(*d*) provision of reference substances and other services;

(*e*) participation in collaborative research developed under the Organization's leadership, including the planning, conduct, monitoring and evaluation of research, as well as promotion of the application of the results of research;

(*f*) training, including research training; and

(*g*) the coordination of activities carried out by several institutions on a given subject.

3.4 A WHO collaborating centre participates on a contractual basis in cooperative programmes supported by the Organization at the country, intercountry, regional, interregional and global levels. It also contributes to increasing technical cooperation with and among countries by providing them with information, services and advice, and by stimulating and supporting research and training.

Designation

3.5 The criteria to be applied in the selection of institutions for designation as a WHO collaborating centre are as follows:

(*a*) the scientific and technical standing of the institution concerned at the national and international levels;

(*b*) the place the institution occupies in the country's health, scientific or educational structures;

(*c*) the quality of its scientific and technical leadership, and the number and qualifications of its staff;

(*d*) the institution's prospective stability in terms of personnel, activity and funding;

(*e*) the working relationship which the institution has developed with other institutions in the country, as well as at the intercountry, regional and global levels;

(*f*) the institution's ability, capacity and readiness to contribute, individually and within networks, to WHO programme activities, whether in support of country programmes or by participating in international cooperative activities;

(*g*) the technical and geographical relevance of the institution and its activities to WHO's programme priorities;

(*h*) the successful completion by the institution of at least two years of collaboration with WHO in carrying out jointly planned activities.

3.6 Regional Directors shall propose institutions for designation as WHO collaborating centres by the Director-General. They shall do so on the basis of preliminary exploration with the institutions and national authorities concerned and with the advice of and on suggestions from the Organization's programme officers responsible, at both global and regional level, for the programmes concerned.

3.7 Regional Directors shall provide the Director-General with appropriate information concerning:

(*a*) the programme requirements to which the prospective centre is expected to respond and the functions it will have to perform;

(*b*) the suitability of the institution concerned, on the basis of the criteria laid down in these regulations and by the Director-General; and (*c*) the government's and institution's agreement to the proposed designation.

3.8 Designation shall be by agreement with the administrative head of the institution after consultation with the national authorities. The designation shall be signified to the institution and the national authorities by the Regional Director concerned.

3.9 After designation, an institution shall be known by the official title "WHO Collaborating Centre", followed by a concise indication of the sphere of activity covered.

3.10 WHO collaborating centres shall be designated for an initial period of four years. The designation is renewable for the same or shorter periods, if warranted by programme requirements and the results of evaluation.

Management

3.11 Collaboration with the centres shall be managed by relevant programme officers in that part of the Organization which initiated the designation process, whether at headquarters or in a region. Collaborating centres, however, shall maintain their technical links with all parts of the Organization relevant to their agreed programme of work.

4. NATIONAL INSTITUTIONS RECOGNIZED BY WHO

4.1 For collaborative activities of such scope or nature as may not warrant the designation of a WHO collaborating centre, the Organization may propose that an institution that is able and willing to participate in such activities with WHO be designated by the national authorities concerned for that purpose.

4.2 Upon designation by the national authorities, such institution shall be formally acknowledged by the Organization as a national institution recognized by WHO. However, no reference to WHO may be included in the title of the institution.

4.3 An agreement shall specify the tasks to be performed by the institution and the technical contributions to be provided by the Organization.

4.4 Official recognition by the Organization shall be for one year and shall be tacitly renewed unless notice is given by either party three months in advance.

4.5 The acknowledgement of such recognition of a national institution by WHO shall be signified to the government and to the institution concerned by the Regional Director. Working technical relationships with the institution shall be developed at regional or headquarters level, as appropriate.

4.6 National institutions recognized by WHO shall be authorized by their respective governments, when such authorization is necessary, to maintain direct working relations with the Organization and with WHO collaborating centres.

5. Other Mechanisms of Collaboration

5.1 Other mechanisms of collaboration with individual experts, expert groups and institutions – for example by contractual technical service agreement – are developed by the Organization in response to particular requirements.

5.2 These mechanisms are mostly based on the very close involvement of individual experts, expert groups and institutions in the definition of programme objectives, the formulation of strategic plans to attain those objectives, the implementation of those plans, and the monitoring of progress.

5.3 The Director-General shall apply to these mechanisms the working procedures he deems most effective, even though these procedures may differ from those provided for in these regulations and those pertaining to expert advisory panels and committees. These mechanisms, however, shall be in general conformity with the principles outlined in these regulations, especially concerning the adequate international and technical distribution of expertise.

5.4 All new developments in the Organization's collaboration with individual experts, expert groups and institutions shall be subjected to the monitoring and evaluation procedures outlined below.

6. Monitoring and Evaluation

6.1 In the development of its individual, collective and institutional mechanisms for expert guidance and support, the Organization must be able to rely on adequate monitoring and evaluation procedures.

6.2 The Director-General shall develop those procedures, using to the full the technical resources of the Secretariat as well as scientific and technical advisory bodies dealing with various aspects of the Organization's programme, in particular the global and regional advisory committees on health research.[1]

---

[1] See footnote 1, p. 116.

6.3 The Director-General shall report to the Executive Board, from time to time, on the results obtained and on any difficulties encountered in giving effect to the above regulations, and shall propose action to ensure their maximum effectiveness.

RULES OF PROCEDURE
OF THE WORLD HEALTH ASSEMBLY[1]

Note: Whenever any of the following terms appear in these Rules, reference shall be as indicated below:

"Constitution" – to the Constitution of the World Health Organization

"Organization" – to the World Health Organization

"Health Assembly" – to the World Health Assembly

"Board" – to the Executive Board

"Members" – to Members of the World Health Organization

"Associate Members" – to Associate Members of the World Health Organization

"Financial period" – to a period of two consecutive calendar years beginning with an even-numbered year.

Preamble

These Rules of Procedure are adopted under the authority of, and are subject to, the Constitution of the World Health Organization. In the event of any conflict between any provision of the Rules and any provision of the Constitution, the Constitution shall prevail.

SESSIONS OF THE HEALTH ASSEMBLY

Rule 1

The Director-General shall convene the Health Assembly to meet annually in regular session at such time and place as the Board shall determine in conformity with the provisions of Articles 14 and 15 of the Constitution.

Rule 2

The Director-General shall convene the Health Assembly to meet in special session, within ninety days of the receipt of any request therefor, made by a majority of the Members and Associate Members of the Organization or by the Board, at such time and place as the Board shall determine.

---

[1] Text adopted by the Eighth World Health Assembly (resolutions WHA8.26 and WHA8.27) and amended by the Tenth, Eleventh, Twelfth, Thirteenth, Fourteenth, Fifteenth, Eighteenth, Twentieth, Twenty-third, Twenty-fifth, Twenty-seventh, Twenty-eighth, Twenty-ninth, Thirtieth, Thirty-first, Thirty-second, Thirty-sixth, Thirty-seventh, Forty-first, Forty-ninth, Fiftieth, and Fifty-seventh World Health Assemblies (resolutions WHA10.44, WHA11.24. WHA11.36, WHA12.39, WHA13.43, WHA14.46, WHA15.50, WHA18.22, WHA20.1, WHA20.30, WHA23.2, WHA25.50, WHA27.17, WHA28.69. WHA29.37, WHA30.1, WHA30.22, WHA31.9, WHA31.13, WHA32.12, WHA32.36, WHA36.16, WHA37.3, WHA41.4, WHA49.7, WHA50.18 and WHA57.8).

Rule 3

Notices convening a regular session of the Health Assembly shall be sent by the Director-General not less than sixty days and notices convening a special session not less than thirty days before the date fixed for the opening of the session, to Members and Associate Members, to representatives of the Board and to all participating intergovernmental and non-governmental organizations admitted into relationship with the Organization invited to be represented at the session.

The Director-General may invite States having made application for membership, territories on whose behalf application for associate membership has been made, and States which have signed but not accepted the Constitution to send observers to sessions of the Health Assembly.

AGENDA OF HEALTH ASSEMBLY SESSIONS

Regular Sessions

Rule 4

The Board shall prepare the provisional agenda of each regular session of the Health Assembly after consideration of proposals submitted by the Director-General. The provisional agenda shall be dispatched together with the notice of convocation mentioned in Rule 3.

Rule 5

The Board shall include in the provisional agenda of each regular session of the Health Assembly *inter alia*:

(*a*) the annual report of the Director-General on the work of the Organization;

(*b*) all items that the Health Assembly has, in a previous session, ordered to be included;

(*c*) any items pertaining to the budget for the next financial period and to reports on the accounts for the preceding year or period;

(*d*) any item proposed by a Member or by an Associate Member;

WHA Rules
of Procedure

(*e*) subject to such preliminary consultation as may be necessary between the Director-General and the Secretary-General of the United Nations, any item proposed by the United Nations;

(*f*) any item proposed by any other organization of the United Nations system with which the Organization has entered into effective relations.

Special Sessions

Rule 6

The Director-General shall draw up the provisional agenda for any special session of the Health Assembly and dispatch it together with the notice of convocation mentioned in Rule 3.

Rule 7

The provisional agenda for each special session shall include only those items proposed in any request by a majority of the Members and Associate Members of the Organization or by the Board for the holding of the session, pursuant to Rule 2.

Regular and Special Sessions

Rule 8

The Director-General shall enter into consultation with the United Nations or the specialized agencies on items, proposed in conformity with these Rules, relating to new activities to be undertaken by the Organization which are of direct concern to such organization or organizations, and shall report to the Health Assembly on the means of achieving co-ordinated use of the resources of the respective organizations.

When such proposals are put forward during the course of a session, the Director-General shall, after such consultation as may be possible with representatives of the United Nations or specialized agencies attending the session, draw the attention of the Health Assembly to the full implications of the proposal.

Rule 9

The Health Assembly shall satisfy itself that adequate consultations have taken place with the organizations concerned in accordance with Rule 8 before taking action on such new activities.

Rule 10

The Director-General shall consult the United Nations and the specialized agencies, as well as Member States, on international conventions or agreements or international regulations proposed for adoption in respect of any provision thereof which affects the activities of such organization or organizations, and shall bring the comments of such organization or organizations to the attention of the Health Assembly together with the comments received from governments.

Rule 11

Unless the Health Assembly decides otherwise in case of urgency, proposals for new activities to be undertaken by the Organization may be placed upon the supplementary agenda of any session only if such proposals are received at least six weeks before the date of the opening of the session, or if the proposal is one which should be referred to another organ of the Organization for examination with a view to deciding whether action by the Organization is desirable.

Rule 12

Subject to the provisions of Rule 11 regarding new activities and to the provisions of Rule 98, a supplementary item may be added to the agenda during any session, if upon the report of the General Committee the Health Assembly so decides, provided that the request for the inclusion of the supplementary item reaches the Organization within six days from the day of the opening of a regular session or within two days from the day of the opening of a special session, both periods being inclusive of the opening day.

Rule 13

The Director-General shall report to the Health Assembly on the technical, administrative and financial implications of all agenda items submitted to the Health Assembly before they are considered by the Health Assembly in plenary meeting. No proposal shall be considered in the absence of such a report unless the Health Assembly decides otherwise in case of urgency.

Rule 14

Copies of all reports and other documents relating to the agenda of any session shall be sent by the Director-General to Members and Associate Members, to representatives of the Board and to participating intergovernmental organizations at the same time as the agenda or as soon thereafter as possible; appropriate reports and documents shall also be sent to non-governmental organizations admitted into relationship with the Organization in the same manner.

Rule 15

The Health Assembly shall not proceed, unless it determines otherwise, to the discussion of any item on the agenda until at least forty-eight hours have elapsed after the documents referred to in Rules 13 and 14 have been made available to delegations.

Nevertheless, the President of the Health Assembly, with the consent of the General Committee, may suspend the application of this Rule. In this case, notice of such suspension shall be given to all delegations and inserted in the *Journal* of the Health Assembly.

SECRETARIAT OF THE HEALTH ASSEMBLY

Rule 16

The Director-General shall be *ex officio* Secretary of the Health Assembly and of any subdivision thereof. He may delegate these functions.

Rule 17

The Director-General shall provide and supervise such secretarial and other staff and facilities as may be required by the Health Assembly.

Rule 18

It shall be the duty of the Secretariat to receive, translate into the working languages of the Health Assembly, and circulate documents, reports and resolutions of the Health Assembly and its committees; to prepare the records of their proceedings; and to perform any other tasks required in connexion with the activities of the Health Assembly or any of its committees.

PLENARY MEETINGS OF THE HEALTH ASSEMBLY

Rule 19

Plenary meetings of the Health Assembly will, unless the Health Assembly decides otherwise, be open to attendance by all delegates, alternates and advisers appointed by Members, in accordance with Articles 10-12 inclusive of the Constitution, by representatives of Associate Members appointed in accordance with Article 8 of the Constitution, and the resolution governing the status of Associate Members, by representatives of the Board, by observers of invited non-Member States and territories on whose behalf application for associate membership has been made, and also by invited representatives of the United Nations and of other participating intergovernmental and non-governmental organizations admitted into relationship with the Organization.

In plenary meetings the chief delegate may designate another delegate who shall have the right to speak and vote in the name of his delegation on any question. Moreover, upon the request of the chief delegate or any delegate so designated by him the President may allow an adviser to speak on any particular point.

Rule 20

Plenary meetings of the Health Assembly shall be held in public unless the Health Assembly decides that exceptional circumstances require that the meeting be held in private. The Health Assembly shall determine the participation at private meetings beyond that of the delegations of Members, the representatives of Associate Members and the representative of the United Nations. Decisions of the Health Assembly taken at a private meeting shall be announced at an early public meeting of the Health Assembly.

Rule 21

Subject to any decision of the Health Assembly, the Director-General shall make appropriate arrangements for the admission of the public and of representatives of the Press and of other information agencies to the plenary meetings of the Health Assembly.

Rule 22

(a) Each Member, Associate Member and participating intergovernmental and invited non-governmental organization shall communicate to the Director-General, if possible fifteen days before the date fixed for the opening of the session of the Health Assembly, the names of its representatives, including all alternates, advisers and secretaries.

(b) The credentials of delegates of Members and of the representatives of Associate Members shall be delivered to the Director-General, if possible not less than one day before the opening of the session of the Health Assembly. Such credentials shall be issued by the Head of State or by the Minister for Foreign Affairs or by the Minister of Health or by any other appropriate authority.

COMMITTEE ON CREDENTIALS

Rule 23

A Committee on Credentials consisting of twelve delegates of as many Members shall be appointed at the beginning of each session by the Health

Assembly on the proposal of the President. This committee shall elect its own officers. It shall examine the credentials of delegates of Members and of the representatives of Associate Members and report to the Health Assembly thereon without delay. Any delegate or representative to whose admission a Member has made objection shall be seated provisionally with the same rights as other delegates or representatives, until the Committee on Credentials has reported and the Health Assembly has given its decision. The Bureau of the Committee shall be empowered to recommend to the Health Assembly on behalf of the Committee the acceptance of the formal credentials of delegates or representatives seated on the basis of provisional credentials already accepted by the Health Assembly.

Meetings of the Committee on Credentials shall be held in private.

COMMITTEE ON NOMINATIONS

Rule 24

The Committee on Nominations of the Health Assembly shall consist of twenty-five delegates of as many Members.

At the beginning of each regular session the President shall submit to the Health Assembly a list consisting of twenty-four Members to comprise, with the President, *ex officio*, the Committee on Nominations. Any Member may propose additions to such list. On the basis of such list, as amended by any additions proposed, a vote shall be taken in accordance with the provisions of those Rules dealing with elections.

Meetings of the Committee on Nominations shall be held in private. The President of the Health Assembly shall preside over meetings of the Committee on Nominations. The President may designate a member of his delegation as his substitute in his capacity as member during a meeting or any part thereof.

Rule 25

The Committee on Nominations, having regard to an equitable geographical distribution and to experience and personal competence, shall propose (*a*) to the Health Assembly from among the delegates nominations for the offices of the President and five vice-presidents of the Health Assembly, for the offices of chairman of each of the main committees, and for the members of the General Committee to be elected under Rule 31, and (*b*) to each of the main committees, set up under Rule 34, nominations from among the delegates for the offices of the two vice-chairmen and rapporteur. The President shall submit an initial list of proposals as set forth above for consideration by the Committee on Nominations. Any member of the Committee may propose additions to such list. On the basis of such list, as amended by any additions proposed, the Committee shall, in accordance with the provisions of Rule 80, determine its list of nominations which shall be forthwith communicated to the Health Assembly or to the main committees respectively.

OFFICERS OF THE HEALTH ASSEMBLY

Rule 26

At each regular session, the Health Assembly, after consideration of the report of the Committee on Nominations, shall elect a President and five Vice-Presidents, who shall hold office until their successors are elected.

Rule 27

In addition to exercising the powers which are conferred upon him elsewhere by these Rules, the President shall declare the opening and closing of each plenary meeting of the session, shall direct the discussions in plenary meetings, ensure observance of these Rules, accord the right to speak, put questions and announce decisions. He shall rule on points of order, and, subject to these Rules, shall control the proceedings at any meeting and shall maintain order thereat. The President may, in the course of the discussion of any item, propose to the Health Assembly the limitation of the time to be allowed to each speaker or the closure of the list of speakers.

Rule 28

The President may appoint one of the Vice-Presidents to take his place during a meeting or any part thereof. A vice-president acting as president shall have the same powers and duties as the President.

If the President is unable to perform his functions during the remainder of the term for which he was elected, a new President shall be elected from among the five Vice-Presidents by the Health Assembly for the unexpired term.

If the President is unable to act in between sessions, one of the Vice-Presidents shall act in his place. The order in which the vice-presidents shall be requested to serve shall be determined by lot at the session at which the election takes place.

Rule 29

The President, or a vice-president acting as president, shall not vote, but he may, if necessary, appoint another delegate or alternate delegate from his delegation to act as the delegate of his government in plenary meetings.

Rule 30

In the event that neither the President nor any vice-president is present at the opening of a session, the Director-General shall preside *ad interim*.

GENERAL COMMITTEE

Rule 31

The General Committee of the Health Assembly shall consist of the President and Vice-Presidents of the Health Assembly, the chairmen of the main committees of the Health Assembly established under Rule 34 and that number of delegates to be elected by the Health Assembly after consideration of the report of the Committee on Nominations as shall provide a total of twenty-five members of the General Committee, provided that no delegation may have more than one representative on the Committee. The President of the Health Assembly shall convene, and preside over, meetings of the General Committee.

Each member of the General Committee may be accompanied by not more than one other member of his delegation.

The President or a vice-president may designate a member of his delegation as his substitute in his capacity as member during a meeting or any part thereof. The chairman of a main committee shall, in the case of absence, designate a vice-chairman of the committee as his substitute, provided that this vice-chairman shall not have the right to vote if he is of the same delegation as another member of the General Committee. Each of the elected delegates shall be entitled to designate another member of his delegation to act as his substitute in the event of his absence from any meeting of the General Committee.

Meetings of the General Committee shall be held in private unless it decides otherwise.

Rule 32 [1]

Meetings of the General Committee may be attended by not more than one member of each delegation to the Health Assembly not represented thereon. Such members may participate without vote in the deliberations of the General Committee if so invited by the Chairman.

Rule 33

In addition to performing such duties as are specified elsewhere in these Rules, the General Committee, in consultation with the Director-General and subject to any decision of the Health Assembly, shall:

(a) decide the time and place of all plenary meetings, of the meetings of the main committees and of all meetings of committees established at plenary meetings during the session. Whenever practicable, the General

---

[1] With regard to this rule, the Eighth World Health Assembly (resolution WHA8.27) adopted the following interpretation:

The attendance of members of delegations under Rule 31 [now Rule 32] is limited to delegations not having one of their members serving on the General Committee.

Committee shall make known a few days in advance the date and hour of meetings of the Health Assembly and of the committees;

(*b*) determine the order of business at each plenary meeting during the session;

(*c*) propose to the Health Assembly the initial allocation to committees of items of the agenda, and if appropriate the deferment of any item to a future Health Assembly;

(*d*) transfer subsequently items of the agenda allocated to committees from one committee to another, if necessary;

(*e*) report on any additions to the agenda under Rule 12;

(*f*) co-ordinate the work of the main committees and all committees established at plenary meetings during the session;

(*g*) fix the date of adjournment of the session; and

(*h*) otherwise facilitate the orderly dispatch of the business of the session.

MAIN COMMITTEES OF THE HEALTH ASSEMBLY

Rule 34

The main committees of the Health Assembly shall be:

(*a*) Committee A – to deal predominantly with programme and budget matters;

(*b*) Committee B – to deal predominantly with administrative, financial and legal matters.

In addition to these two main committees, the Health Assembly may establish such other main committees as it may consider necessary.

The Health Assembly, after consideration of the recommendations of the Board and the General Committee, shall allocate items of the agenda to the two main committees in such a way as to provide an appropriate balance in the work of these committees.

The chairmen of these main committees shall be elected by the Health Assembly after consideration of the report of the Committee on Nominations.

Rule 35

Each delegation shall be entitled to be represented on each main committee by one of its members. He may be accompanied at meetings of the committee by one or more other members, who may be accorded permission to speak but shall not vote.

Rule 36

Each main committee shall, after consideration of the report of the Committee on Nominations, elect two Vice-Chairmen and a Rapporteur.

Rule 37

To facilitate the conduct of its business, a main committee may designate an additional vice-chairman *ad interim* if its chairman and vice-chairmen are not available.

Rule 38

The chairman of each main committee shall have in relation to the meetings of the committee concerned the same powers and duties as the President of the Health Assembly in relation to plenary meetings.

Rule 39

Meetings of the main committees and their sub-committees shall be held in public unless the committee or sub-committee concerned decides otherwise.

Rule 40

Any main committee may set up such sub-committees or other subdivisions as it considers necessary.[1]

Rule 41

The members of each sub-committee shall be appointed by the main committee concerned upon the proposal of its chairman. A member of a sub-committee who is unable to be present at any meeting may be represented by another member of his delegation.

Each sub-committee shall elect its own officers.

OTHER COMMITTEES OF THE HEALTH ASSEMBLY

Rule 42

The Health Assembly may appoint, or authorize the appointment of, any other committee or subdivision which it deems necessary.

RAPPORTEURS

Rule 43

Any committee, sub-committee or other subdivision may appoint from among its members one or more rapporteurs as required.

---

[1] The Executive Board has recommended that the establishment of working parties in the Health Assembly should be restricted to the following purposes:
   (1) to formulate a conclusion on which substantial agreement has been reached (whether unanimously or by an evident majority);
   (2) to make clear and state the issues that are before the committee for decision;
   (3) to provide a committee with an expert opinion relevant to its discussions.

(*Off. Rec. Wld Hlth Org.*, **33**, 30)

PARTICIPATION OF REPRESENTATIVES OF THE EXECUTIVE BOARD

Rule 44

The Board shall be represented at the Health Assembly by such person or persons serving on the Board as the Board may determine. If any such person is prevented from attending the Health Assembly, the Chairman of the Board shall appoint from amongst the members of the Board a representative to replace him.

Rule 45

Representatives of the Board may attend plenary meetings and meetings of the General Committee and main committees of the Health Assembly. They may participate without vote in their deliberations on the invitation or with the consent of the President of the Health Assembly or the chairman of the committee as the case may be.

PARTICIPATION OF REPRESENTATIVES OF ASSOCIATE MEMBERS
AND OF INTERGOVERNMENTAL AND NON-GOVERNMENTAL
ORGANIZATIONS AND OF OBSERVERS OF NON-MEMBER STATES
AND TERRITORIES

Rule 46

Representatives of Associate Members may participate equally with Members in meetings of the Health Assembly and of its main committees except that they shall not hold office nor shall they have the right to vote.

They may participate equally with Members in other committees, subcommittees or other subdivisions of the Health Assembly except the General Committee, the Committee on Credentials and the Committee on Nominations.

Rule 47

Observers of invited non-Member States and territories on whose behalf application for associate membership has been made may attend any open meetings of the Health Assembly or any of its main committees. They may, upon the invitation of the President, and with the consent of the Health Assembly or committee, make a statement on the subject under discussion.

Such observers shall have access to non-confidential documents and to such other documents as the Director-General may see fit to make available. They may submit memoranda to the Director-General, who shall determine the nature and scope of their circulation.

Rule 48

Subject to the terms of any agreement, representatives of the United Nations and of other intergovernmental organizations with which the

Organization has established effective relations under Article 70 of the Constitution, may participate without vote in the deliberations of meetings of the Health Assembly and its main committees. Such representatives may also attend and participate without vote in the deliberations of the meetings of sub-committees or other subdivisions if so invited.

They shall have access to non-confidential documents and to such other documents as the Director-General may see fit to make available. They may submit memoranda to the Director-General, who shall determine the nature and scope of their circulation.

Rule 49

Representatives of non-governmental organizations with which arrangements for consultation and co-operation have been made, in accordance with Article 71 of the Constitution, may be invited to attend plenary meetings and meetings of the main committees of the Health Assembly and to participate without vote therein in accordance with those arrangements, when invited to do so by the President of the Health Assembly or by the chairman of a main committee, respectively.

CONDUCT OF BUSINESS AT PLENARY MEETINGS

Rule 50

Formal proposals relating to items of the agenda may be introduced at plenary meetings up to the date on which all items of the agenda have been allocated to committees or until fourteen days after the opening of the session, whichever date is the earlier.

Rule 51

All such proposals shall be referred to the committee to which the item of the agenda has been allocated. Thereafter all proposals relating to items of the agenda must be introduced in the first instance in the committee concerned or in an appropriate sub-committee thereof.

Rule 52

Proposals and amendments shall normally be introduced in writing and handed to the Director-General, who shall circulate copies to the delegations. Except as may be decided otherwise by the Health Assembly, no proposal shall be discussed or put to the vote at any meeting of the Health Assembly unless copies of it have been circulated to all delegations at least two days previously. The President may, however, permit the discussion and consideration of amendments, even though they have not been circulated or have only been circulated the same day.

Rule 53

The reports of all committees shall be submitted by these committees to a plenary meeting. Such reports, including draft resolutions, shall be distributed, in so far as practicable, at least twenty-four hours in advance of the plenary meeting at which they are to be considered. Such reports, including draft resolutions annexed thereto, shall not be read aloud in the plenary meetings unless the President decides otherwise.

Rule 54

A majority of the Members represented at the session shall constitute a quorum for the conduct of business at plenary meetings of the Health Assembly.

Rule 55

No delegate may address the Health Assembly without having previously obtained the permission of the President. The President shall call upon speakers in the order in which they signify their desire to speak. The President may call a speaker to order if his remarks are not relevant to the subject under discussion.

Rule 56

The Director-General or a member of the Secretariat designated by him may at any time make either oral or written statements to the Health Assembly or to any of its committees or subdivisions concerning any question under consideration.

Rule 57

The Health Assembly may limit the time allowed to each speaker.

Rule 58

During the discussion of any matter a delegate or a representative of an Associate Member may rise to a point of order[1] and the point of order shall be immediately decided by the President. A delegate or a representative of an Associate Member may appeal against the ruling of the President, in which case the appeal shall immediately be put to the vote. A delegate or a

---

[1] For description of the concept of a point of order, see p. 151.

representative of an Associate Member rising to a point of order may not speak on the substance of the matter under discussion, but on the point of order only.

Rule 59

The right of reply shall be accorded by the President to any delegate or representative of an Associate Member who requests it. Delegates and representatives of Associate Members should in exercising this right attempt to be as brief as possible and preferably deliver their statements at the end of the meeting at which this right is requested.

Rule 60

During the course of a debate the President may announce the list of speakers and, with the consent of the Health Assembly, declare the list closed. He may, however, accord the right of reply to any member if in his opinion a speech delivered after he has declared the list closed makes this desirable.

Rule 61

During the discussion of any matter, a delegate or a representative of an Associate Member may move the suspension or the adjournment of the meeting. Such motions shall not be debated, but shall immediately be put to a vote.

For the purpose of these Rules "suspension of the meeting" means the temporary postponement of the business of the meeting and "adjournment of the meeting" the termination of all business until another meeting is called.

Rule 62

During the discussion of any matter a delegate or a representative of an Associate Member may move the adjournment of the debate on the item under discussion. In addition to the proposer of the motion, one speaker may speak in favour of, and one against, the motion, after which the motion to adjourn the debate shall be immediately put to the vote.

Rule 63

A delegate or a representative of an Associate Member may at any time move the closure of the debate on the item under discussion whether or not any other delegate or representative of an Associate Member has signified his wish to speak. If request is made for permission to speak against closure, it may be accorded to not more than two speakers, after which the motion shall be immediately put to the vote. If the Health Assembly decides in favour of closure, the President shall declare the debate closed. The Health Assembly shall thereafter vote only on the one or more proposals moved before the closure.

Rule 64

The following motions shall have precedence in the following order over all other proposals or motions before the meeting, except a point of order:

(*a*) to suspend the meeting;

(*b*) to adjourn the meeting;

(*c*) to adjourn the debate on the item under discussion; and

(*d*) for the closure of the debate on the item under discussion.

Rule 65

Subject to Rule 64, any motion calling for a decision on the competence of the Health Assembly to adopt a proposal submitted to it shall be put to the vote before a vote is taken on the proposal in question.

Rule 66

A delegate or a representative of an Associate Member may move that parts of a proposal or of an amendment shall be voted on separately. If objection is made to the request for division, the motion for division shall be voted upon. Permission to speak on the motion for division shall be given only to two speakers in favour and two speakers against. If the motion for division is carried, those parts of the proposal or of the amendment which are subsequently approved shall be put to the vote as a whole. If all operative parts of the proposal or the amendment have been rejected, the proposal or the amendment shall be considered to have been rejected as a whole.

Rule 67

When an amendment to a proposal is moved, the amendment shall be voted on first. When two or more amendments to a proposal are moved, the Health Assembly shall first vote on the amendment deemed by the President to be furthest removed in substance from the original proposal, and then on the amendment next removed therefrom, and so on, until all the amendments have been put to the vote. Where, however, the adoption of one amendment necessarily implies the rejection of another amendment, the latter amendment shall not be put to the vote. If one or more amendments are adopted, the amended proposal shall then be voted upon. If an amendment to a proposal has been accepted by the original proposer, such an amendment shall be deemed to be an integral part of the original proposal and no separate vote shall be required thereon. A motion is considered an amendment to a proposal if it merely adds to, deletes from or revises part of that proposal. A motion which constitutes a substitution for a proposal shall be considered as a proposal.

Rule 68

If two or more proposals are moved, the Health Assembly shall first vote on the proposal deemed by the President to be furthest removed in substance from the proposal first presented and then on the proposal next removed therefrom, and so on, until all the proposals have been put to the vote, unless the result of a vote on a proposal makes unnecessary any other voting on the proposal or proposals still outstanding.

Rule 69

A motion may be withdrawn by its proposer at any time before voting on it has commenced, provided that the motion has not been amended or, if amended, that the proposer of the amendment agrees to the withdrawal. A motion thus withdrawn may be reintroduced by any delegate.

Rule 70

When a proposal has been adopted or rejected, it may not be reconsidered at the same session unless the Health Assembly, by a two-thirds majority of the Members present and voting, so decides. Permission to speak on a motion to reconsider shall be accorded only to two speakers opposing the motion, after which it shall immediately be put to a vote. The correction of a clerical or arithmetical error in any document concerning a proposal which has already been adopted shall not be considered as requiring the reopening of the debate on such proposal by a two-thirds majority vote.

VOTING IN PLENARY MEETINGS

Rule 71

Each Member shall have one vote in the Health Assembly. For the purposes of these Rules, the phrase "Members present and voting" means

Members casting a valid affirmative or negative vote. Members abstaining from voting are considered as not voting.

Rule 72

Decisions by the Health Assembly on important questions shall be made by a two thirds majority of the Members present and voting. These questions shall include: the adoption of conventions or agreements; the approval of agreements bringing the Organization into relation with the United Nations and with intergovernmental organizations and agencies in accordance with Articles 69, 70 and 72 of the Constitution; amendments to the Constitution; appointment of the Director-General; decisions on the amount of the effective working budget; and decisions to suspend the voting privileges and services of a Member under Article 7 of the Constitution.

Rule 73

Except as stipulated otherwise in these Rules, decisions on other questions, including the determination of additional categories of questions to be decided by a two-thirds majority, shall be made by a majority of the Members present and voting.

Rule 74

The Health Assembly shall normally vote by show of hands, except that any delegate may request a roll-call, which shall then be taken in the English or French alphabetical order of the names of the Members, in alternate years. The name of the Member to vote first shall be determined by lot.

Rule 75

The vote of each Member participating in any roll-call shall be inserted in the record of the meeting.

Rule 76

After the President has announced the beginning of voting, no delegate shall interrupt the voting except on a point of order in connexion with the actual conduct of voting.

Rule 77

After the voting has been completed, a delegate may make a brief statement, consisting solely of an explanation of vote. A sponsor of a proposal shall not speak in explanation of vote thereon, except if it has been amended.

Rule 78

In addition to the cases provided for elsewhere by these Rules, the Health Assembly may vote on any matter by secret ballot if it has previously so decided by a majority of the Members present and voting, provided that no secret ballot may be taken on budgetary questions.

A decision under this Rule by the Health Assembly whether or not to vote by secret ballot may only be taken by a show of hands; if the Assembly has decided to vote on a particular question by secret ballot, no other mode of voting may be requested or decided upon.

Rule 79

When the Health Assembly votes by secret ballot, the ballot itself and the check of the number of ballot papers shall take place in plenary meeting. Unless the Health Assembly determines otherwise the counting of votes shall take place in a separate room to which delegations shall have access. This counting shall take place under the supervision of the President or of one of the Vice-Presidents of the Health Assembly. The Health Assembly may proceed with its work during the period before the results of the ballot can be announced.

Rule 80

Elections shall normally be held by secret ballot.[1] Subject to the provisions of Rule 110, and in the absence of any objection, the Health Assembly may decide to proceed without taking a ballot on an agreed candidate or list of candidates. Where a ballot is required, two tellers appointed by the President from among the delegations present shall assist in the counting of votes.

Rule 81

When only one person or Member is to be elected and no candidate obtains in the first ballot the majority required, a second ballot shall be taken which shall be restricted to the two candidates obtaining the largest number of votes. If in the second ballot the votes are equally divided, the President shall decide between the candidates by drawing lots.

Rule 82

When two or more elective places are to be filled at one time under the same conditions, those candidates obtaining in the first ballot the majority required shall be elected. If the number of candidates obtaining such majority is less than the number of persons or Members to be elected, there shall

---

[1] For Guiding Principles for the Conduct of Elections by Secret Ballot, see p. 150.

be additional ballots to fill the remaining places, the ballots being restricted to the candidates obtaining the greatest number of votes in the previous ballot to a number not more than twice the places remaining to be filled; provided that, after the third inconclusive ballot, votes may be cast for any eligible person or Member. If three such unrestricted ballots are inconclusive, the next three ballots shall be restricted to the candidates who obtained the greatest number of votes in the third of the unrestricted ballots, to a number not more than twice the places remaining to be filled, and the following three ballots thereafter shall be unrestricted, and so on until all the places have been filled.

Rule 83

In an election each Member, unless he abstains, shall vote for that number of candidates equal to the number of elective places to be filled. Any ballot paper on which there are more or fewer names than there are elective places to be filled shall be null and void.

Rule 84

If during an election one or more elective places cannot be filled by reason of an equal number of votes having been obtained by two or more candidates, a ballot shall be held among such candidates to determine which of them will be elected. This procedure may be repeated if necessary. If the votes are equally divided on a matter other than an election the proposal shall be regarded as not adopted.

CONDUCT OF BUSINESS AND VOTING IN COMMITTEES AND SUB-COMMITTEES

Rule 85

Subject to any decision of the Health Assembly, the procedure governing the conduct of business and voting by committees shall conform as far as practicable to the Rules relative to the conduct of business and voting in plenary meetings. One-third of the members of a committee shall constitute a quorum. The presence of a majority of a committee shall, however, be required for a question to be put to a vote.

Rule 86

The chairman of each sub-committee shall apply the Rules applicable to committees to the work of such sub-committee only in so far as he considers it advisable with a view to expediting the dispatch of business.

Languages [1]

Rule 87

Arabic, Chinese, English, French, Russian and Spanish shall be both the official and the working languages of the Health Assembly.

Rule 88

Speeches made in an official language shall be interpreted into the other official languages.

Rule 89

Any delegate or any representative of an Associate Member or any representative of the Board may speak in a language other than the official languages. In this case he shall himself provide for interpretation into one of the official languages. Interpretation into the other official languages by interpreters of the Secretariat may be based on the interpretation given in the first such language.

Rule 90

Verbatim and summary records and the *Journal* of the Health Assembly shall be drawn up in the working languages.

Rule 91

All resolutions, recommendations and other formal decisions of the Health Assembly shall be made available in the working languages.

Records of the Health Assembly

Rule 92

Verbatim records of all plenary meetings and summary records of the meetings of the General Committee and of committees and sub-committees shall be made by the Secretariat. Unless otherwise expressly decided by the committee concerned, no record shall be made of the proceedings of the Committee on Nominations or of the Committee on Credentials other than the report presented by the Committee to the Health Assembly.

---

[1] See resolution WHA31.13.

Rule 93

The summary records referred to in Rule 92 shall be sent as soon as possible to delegations, to representatives of Associate Members and to the representatives of the Board, who shall inform the Secretariat in writing not later than forty-eight hours thereafter of any corrections they wish to have made.

Rule 94

As soon as possible after the close of each session, copies of all verbatim and summary records, resolutions, recommendations and other formal decisions adopted by the Health Assembly shall be transmitted by the Director-General to Members and Associate Members, to the United Nations and to all specialized agencies with which the Organization has entered into effective relations. The records of private meetings shall be transmitted to the participants only.

Rule 95

Verbatim and summary records of public meetings and the reports of all committees and sub-committees shall be published.

Rule 96

The Director-General shall issue for the convenience of participating delegations and organizations, in the form of a daily *Journal* of the session, such summary account of the proceedings of plenary meetings, committees and sub-committees as he may consider practicable.

BUDGET AND FINANCE

Rule 97

The Health Assembly shall:

(*a*) adopt the budget authorizing expenditure for the next financial period after consideration of the Director-General's budget estimates and the Board's recommendations thereon;

(*b*) consider and approve supplementary estimates for the current financial period if and as necessary;

(*c*) examine reports of the auditor on the accounts of receipts and expenditures for the preceding financial year or period and take such action thereon as may be appropriate;

(*d*) consider the report of the Director-General on the payment of Members' and Associate Members' contributions.

Rule 98

No proposal for a review of the apportionment of the contributions among Members and Associate Members for the time being in force shall be placed on the agenda unless it has been communicated to Members and Associate Members at least ninety days before the opening of the session, or unless the Board has recommended such review.

Rule 99

Except in so far as there is an express provision to the contrary in the Financial Regulations, the procedure for the consideration of financial matters shall be governed by these Rules.

EXECUTIVE BOARD

Rule 100

At each regular session of the Health Assembly, the Members entitled to designate persons to serve on the Board shall be elected in accordance with Articles 18(*b*), 24 and 25 of the Constitution.

Rule 101

At the commencement of each regular session of the Health Assembly the President shall request Members desirous of putting forward suggestions regarding the annual election of those Members to be entitled to designate a person to serve on the Board to place their suggestions before the General Committee. Such suggestions shall reach the Chairman of the General Committee not later than twenty-four hours after the President has made the announcement in accordance with this Rule.

Rule 102

The General Committee, having regard to the provisions of Chapter VI of the Constitution, to Rule 100, to the suggestions placed before it by Members, and to the candidatures put forward by the members of the General Committee during its meeting, shall by secret ballot draw up a list consisting of at most fifteen Members and at least the same number of

Members as the number of seats to be filled. This list shall be transmitted to the Health Assembly at least twenty-four hours before the Health Assembly convenes for the purpose of the annual election of Members to be entitled to designate a person to serve on the Board.

The General Committee shall recommend in such list to the Health Assembly the Members which, in the Committee's opinion, would provide, if elected, a balanced distribution of the Board as a whole.

Members included in such list other than the Members which, in the Committee's opinion, would provide, if elected, a balanced distribution of the Board as a whole may withdraw their candidatures from the list by notification to the President not later than the closure of working hours on the day preceding the annual election by the Health Assembly of Members to be entitled to designate a person to serve on the Board. Any such withdrawal shall be published in the *Journal* of the Health Assembly and announced by the President prior to the commencement of voting.

Rule 103

Subject to the provisions of Rule 80, the Health Assembly shall elect by secret ballot from among the Members nominated in accordance with the provisions of Rule 102 the Members to be entitled to designate persons to serve on the Board. Those candidates obtaining the majority required shall be elected. If after five such ballots one or more seats remain to be filled no further ballot shall be taken and the General Committee shall be requested to submit nominations for candidates for the seats remaining to be filled, in accordance with Rule 102, the number of candidates so nominated not exceeding twice the number of seats remaining to be filled. Additional ballots shall be taken for the seats remaining to be filled and those candidates obtaining the majority required shall be elected.

If after three such ballots one or more seats remain to be filled, the candidate obtaining in the third ballot the least number of votes shall be eliminated and a further ballot taken, and so on until all the seats have been filled.

In any ballots taken under the provisions of this Rule no nominations other than those made in accordance with the provisions of Rule 102 and this Rule shall be considered.

Rule 104

Should a Member, entitled by a previous election to designate a person to serve on the Board, for any reason surrender such right before the expiration of the term for which elected, or under the provisions of Rule 107 have forfeited such right, the Health Assembly, at a regular session, shall elect another Member to be entitled to designate a person for the remainder of the period to which the Member having so surrendered or forfeited its right would otherwise have been entitled. Such election shall, *mutatis mutandis*, be subject to Rules 83, 84 and 101 to 103, provided that not more than twice the number of candidates for the number of seats vacant shall be nominated and provided that such elections shall precede the annual election of the Members entitled to designate a person to serve on the Board in accordance with Rule 100.

Rule 105

The term of office of each Member entitled to designate a person to serve on the Board shall begin immediately after the closing of the session of the Health Assembly at which the Member concerned is elected and shall end immediately after the closing of the session of the Health Assembly during which the Member is replaced.

Rule 106

When a person designated to serve on the Board is prevented from attending a meeting of the Board, the Member concerned may designate an alternate to serve in his place for such a meeting, with the same status as the person in whose place he is serving.

Rule 107

Should the person designated by any Member to serve on the Board, in accordance with the provisions of Rules 100 and 106, fail to attend two consecutive sessions of the Board, that fact shall be reported by the Director-General to the next session of the Health Assembly and, unless the Health Assembly decides otherwise, that Member shall be deemed to have forfeited its right to designate a person to serve on the Board.

THE DIRECTOR-GENERAL

Rule 108

In pursuance of Article 31 of the Constitution, the Director-General shall be appointed by the Health Assembly on the nomination of the Board and on such terms as the Health Assembly may determine, subject to the provisions of Rules 109 to 112 inclusive. The term of office of the Director-General shall be five years, and he or she shall be eligible for reappointment once only.

Rule 109

Whenever the office of Director-General is vacant or notice is received of a pending vacancy, the Board shall, at its next meeting, make a nomination which shall be submitted to the next session of the Health Assembly. It shall submit at the same time a draft contract establishing the terms and conditions of appointment, salary and other emoluments attached to the office.

Rule 110

The Health Assembly shall consider the Board's nomination at a private meeting and shall come to a decision by secret ballot.

Rule 111

Should the Health Assembly reject the Board's nomination, the Board shall submit a fresh proposal as soon as circumstances permit, with due regard to the desirability of disposing of the matter before the conclusion of the relevant session of the Health Assembly.

Rule 112

The contract of appointment shall be approved by the Health Assembly and shall be signed jointly by the Director-General and by the President of the Health Assembly acting in the name of the Organization.

Rule 113

In any case where the Director-General is unable to perform the functions of his office, or in the case of a vacancy in such office, the senior officer of the Secretariat shall serve as Acting Director-General, subject to any decision by the Board.

Rule 114

In addition to exercising the functions conferred upon him by the Constitution as chief technical and administrative officer of the Organization, the Director-General, subject to the authority of the Board, shall perform such duties as are specified elsewhere in these Rules and in the Financial Regulations and Staff Regulations and as may be assigned to him by the Health Assembly or by the Board.

ADMISSION OF MEMBERS AND ASSOCIATE MEMBERS

Rule 115

Applications made by a State for admission to membership or applications made by a Member or other authority having the responsibility for the international relations of a territory or group of territories on behalf of such territory or group of territories for admission to associate membership in the Organization shall, in pursuance of Articles 6 and 8 of the Constitution, be addressed to the Director-General and shall be transmitted immediately by him to Members.

Any such application shall be placed on the agenda of the next session of the Health Assembly provided the application reaches the Director-General at least thirty days before the opening of such session.

An application for membership made by a State formerly an Associate Member may be received at any time by the Health Assembly.

Rule 116

The approval by the Health Assembly of any request for membership shall be immediately communicated to the State which has submitted it. Such State, in accordance with Article 79 of the Constitution, may then deposit with the Secretary-General of the United Nations a formal instrument of acceptance of the Constitution and shall become a Member from the date of such deposit.

Rule 117

The approval by the Health Assembly of any request for associate membership by a Member or other authority having responsibility for the international relations of a territory or group of territories on behalf of such territory or group of territories shall be communicated immediately to the Member or other authority which has submitted the request. Such Member or other authority shall give notice to the Organization of acceptance on behalf of the Associate Member of associate membership. The territory or group of territories shall become an Associate Member from the date on which such notice is received.

Rule 118

A Member or other authority responsible for the international relations of an Associate Member, who gives notice of acceptance on behalf of such Associate Member under Rule 117, shall include in such notice a statement that the Member or other authority assumes the responsibility for ensuring the application of Articles 66 to 68 of the Constitution with regard to that Associate Member.

AMENDMENT OF THE CONSTITUTION

Rule 119

In pursuance of Article 73 of the Constitution, the texts of proposed amendments to the Constitution shall be communicated to the Director-General in such time as will permit of the transmission of copies thereof by the Director-General to Members not later than six months before the opening day of the session of the Health Assembly at which they are intended to be considered.

Rule 120

Members accepting amendments adopted by the Health Assembly in accordance with Article 73 of the Constitution shall effect their acceptance by depositing a formal instrument with the Secretary-General of the United Nations.

AMENDMENT AND SUSPENSION OF RULES OF PROCEDURE

Rule 121

Amendments of, or additions to, these Rules may be adopted at any plenary meeting of the Health Assembly, provided that the Health Assembly has received and considered a report thereon by an appropriate committee.

Rule 122

Subject to the provisions of the Constitution, any of these Rules may be suspended at any plenary meeting of the Health Assembly, provided that notice of the intention to propose suspension has been communicated to delegations not less than twenty-four hours before the meeting at which the proposal is to be made.

Guiding Principles for the Conduct of Elections by Secret Ballot

1. Before voting begins, the President shall hand to the two tellers appointed by him the list of Members entitled to vote and the list of candidates. For the elections of Members entitled to designate persons to serve on the Executive Board or of the Director-General, the list of candidates shall include only those nominations submitted to the World Health Assembly in accordance with the procedure laid down in Rules 102 and 110 respectively of the Rules of Procedure of the World Health Assembly.

2. The Secretariat shall distribute a ballot paper to each delegation. Every ballot paper shall be of the same size and colour without distinguishing marks.

3. The tellers shall satisfy themselves that the ballot box is empty and, having locked it, shall hand the key to the President.

4. Members shall be called in turn to vote in the required alphabetical order of their names,[1] beginning with the name of a Member which shall have been drawn by lot. The call shall be made in English, French, Russian and Spanish.

5. The secretary of the meeting and the tellers shall record each Member's vote by marking the margin of the list of Members entitled to vote opposite to the name of the Member in question.

6. At the conclusion of the calling of Members, the President shall ensure that all the Members present and entitled to vote have been called. He shall then declare the voting closed and announce that the votes are to be counted.

7. When the ballot box has been opened, the tellers shall count the number of ballot papers. If the number is not equal to that of the voters, the President shall declare the vote invalid and another ballot shall be held.

8. Where the counting of votes takes place outside the Assembly Hall, the ballot papers shall be returned to the ballot box which shall be taken by the tellers to the room where the votes are to be counted.

9. One of the tellers shall then read aloud the names which are on the ballot paper. The number of votes obtained by each of the candidates mentioned shall be written opposite their names by the other teller on a document drawn up for this purpose.

10. A ballot paper on which no names are written or which bears the word "abstention" shall be considered as signifying an abstention.

11. The following shall be considered null and void:

   (*a*) ballot papers on which there are more or fewer names than there are elective places to be filled or on which the name of any candidate appears more than once;

   (*b*) ballot papers in which the voters have revealed their identity, in particular by apposing their signature or mentioning the name of the Member they represent;

---

[1] Under Rule 74 of the Rules of Procedure of the World Health Assembly (see p. 139).

(*c*) where the Rules of Procedure so require, ballot papers bearing the names of candidates other than those nominated in accordance with the provisions of those Rules.

12. When the counting of the votes is completed, the tellers shall indicate the results in a document drawn up for this purpose, which they shall sign and hand to the President. The latter, in plenary meeting, shall announce the results in the following order: number of Members entitled to vote; number absent; number of abstentions; number of ballot papers null and void; number of Members present and voting; number required for a majority; names of candidates and the number of votes secured by each of them, in descending order of the number of votes.

13. For the purposes of these provisions, the following definitions shall apply:

(*a*) "Absent" – Members entitled to vote but whose representatives are not present at the meeting at which the secret ballot takes place;

(*b*) "Number of Members present and voting" – the difference between the number of Members with the right to vote and the total number of absentees, abstentions and invalid ballot papers.

14. The President shall declare elected candidates who have obtained the required majority.

15. The list signed by the tellers and on which the results of the vote have been recorded shall constitute the official record of the count of the ballot and shall be retained in the Organization's files. The ballot papers shall be destroyed immediately after the declaration of the results of the ballot.

Description of the Concept of a Point of Order

(*a*) A point of order is basically an intervention directed to the presiding officer, requesting him to make use of some power inherent in his office or specifically given him under the Rules of Procedure. It may, for example, relate to the manner in which the debate is conducted, to the maintenance of order, to the observance of the Rules of Procedure, or to the way in which presiding officers exercise the powers conferred upon them by the Rules. Under a point of order, a delegate or a representative of an Associate Member may request the presiding officer to apply a certain Rule of Procedure or he may question the way in which the officer applies the Rule. Thus, within the scope of the Rules of Procedure, delegates or representatives are enabled to direct the attention of the presiding officer to violations or misapplications of the Rules by other delegates or representatives or by the presiding officer himself. A point of order has precedence over any other matter, including procedural motions (Rules 58 and 64).

(*b*) Points of order raised under Rule 58 involve questions necessitating a ruling by the presiding officer, subject to possible appeal. They are therefore distinct from the procedural motions provided for in Rules 61 to 64, which can be decided only by a vote and on which more than one motion may be entertained at the same time, Rule 64 laying down the precedence of such motions. They are also distinct from requests for information or clarification, or from remarks relating to material arrangements (seating, interpretation system, temperature of the room), documents, translations, etc., which – while they may have to be dealt with by the presiding officer – do not require rulings from him. However, in established practice, a delegate or a representative of an Associate Member intending to submit a procedural motion or to seek information or clarification often rises to "a point of order" as a means of obtaining the floor. The latter usage, which is based on practical grounds, should not be confused with the raising of points of order under Rule 58.

(*c*) Under Rule 58, a point of order must be immediately decided by the presiding officer in accordance with the Rules of Procedure; any appeal arising therefrom must also be put immediately to the vote. It follows that, as a general rule:

(i) Neither a point of order, nor any appeal arising from a ruling thereon, is debatable;

(ii) No point of order on the same or a different subject can be permitted until the initial point of order and any appeal arising therefrom have been disposed of.

Nevertheless, both the presiding officer and delegations may request information or clarification regarding a point of order. In addition, the presiding officer may, if he considers it necessary, request an expression of views from delegations on a point of order before giving his ruling; in the exceptional cases in which this practice is resorted to, the presiding officer should terminate the exchange of views and give his ruling as soon as he is ready to announce that ruling.

(d) Rule 58 provides that a delegate or a representative of an Associate Member rising to a point of order may not speak on the substance of the matter under discussion. Consequently, the purely procedural nature of points of order calls for brevity. The presiding officer is responsible for ensuring that statements made on a point of order are in conformity with the present description.

RULES OF PROCEDURE OF THE EXECUTIVE BOARD OF THE WORLD HEALTH ORGANIZATION[1]

MEMBERSHIP AND ATTENDANCE

Rule 1

The Executive Board (hereinafter referred to as the "Board") shall, in accordance with Chapter VI of the Constitution of the World Health Organization (hereinafter referred to as the "Organization") and Rules 100-107 of the Rules of Procedure of the World Health Assembly (hereinafter referred to as the "Health Assembly") consist of and be attended by the persons (hereinafter referred to as the "members") duly designated to serve on the Board.

Rule 2

Each State Member entitled to designate a person to serve on the Board shall inform the Director-General in writing of the names of the person designated and of any alternate and adviser. The Director-General shall similarly be informed of any change in such designation.

Rule 3

All Member States not represented on the Board and Associate Members may designate a representative who shall have the right to participate without vote in the deliberations of meetings of the Board and of committees of limited membership (as defined in Rule 16) established by it.

The cost of representation under this Rule shall be borne by the Member State or Associate Member concerned.

Representatives of Member States and Associate Members participating in meetings under this Rule shall have the following rights: (*a*) the right to speak after members of the Board; (*b*) the right to make proposals, and amendments to proposals, which shall be considered by the Board only if seconded by a Board member; and (*c*) the right of reply.

---

[1] Text adopted by the Executive Board at its seventeenth session (resolution EB17.R63) and amended at its twentieth, twenty-first, twenty-second, twenty-eighth, thirty-first, thirty-seventh, fifty-third, fifty-seventh, ninety-seventh, 102nd and 112th sessions (resolutions EB20.R24, EB21.R52, EB22.R11, EB28.R21, EB31.R15, EB37.R24, EB53.R29, EB53.R37, EB57.R38, EB97.R10, EB102.R1 and EB112.R1).

Rule 4

Subject to the terms of any relevant agreement, representatives of the United Nations and of other intergovernmental organizations with which the Organization has established effective relations under Article 70 of the Constitution may participate without vote in the deliberations of meetings of the Board and its committees. Such representatives may also attend and participate without vote in the deliberations of the meetings of sub-committees or other subdivisions if so invited.

Representatives of nongovernmental organizations in official relations with the Organization may participate in the deliberations of the Board as is provided for participation in the Health Assembly in the "Principles governing relations between the World Health Organization and nongovernmental organizations".[1]

SESSIONS

Rule 5

The Board shall hold at least two sessions a year. It shall determine at each session the time and place of its next session.

Notices convening the Board shall be sent by the Director-General eight weeks before the commencement of a regular session to the members of the Board, to Member States and Associate Members and to the organizations referred to in Rule 4 invited to be represented at the session.

Documents for the session shall be dispatched by the Director-General not less than six weeks before the commencement of a regular session of the Board. They shall, at the same time, be made available in electronic form in the working languages of the Board on the Internet site of the Organization.

Documents for the session should conform to the functions of the Board and contain the information required by Rule 18 and clear recommendations for Board action.

Rule 6

The Director-General shall also convene the Board at the joint request of any ten members, addressed to him in writing and stating the reason for the request. In this case the Board shall be convened within thirty days following receipt of the request and the session shall be held at headquarters unless the Director-General, in consultation with the Chairman, determines otherwise. The agenda of such a session shall be limited to the questions having necessitated that session.

If events occur requiring immediate action under Article 28(*i*) of the Constitution the Director-General may, in consultation with the Chairman,

---

[1] See p. 81.

convene the Board in a special session and shall fix the date and determine the place of the session.

Rule 7

Attendance at meetings of the Board shall, in addition to members of the Board, their alternates and advisers, be as follows:

(*a*) public meetings: Member States not represented on the Board, Associate Members, representatives of the United Nations and other organizations identified in Rule 4 and members of the public; or

(*b*) open meetings: Member States not represented on the Board and Associate Members and the Secretariat; or

(*c*) restricted meetings, held for a specific purpose and under exceptional circumstances: essential Secretariat staff, and such others as may be decided by the Board.

Meetings of the Board related to the nomination of the Director-General as provided for in Rule 52, and for the appointment of the Regional Directors, shall be as provided in subparagraph (*b*) above, except that only one representative of each Member State not represented on the Board and of each Associate Member may attend without the right to participate, and that no official record shall be made.

AGENDA

Rule 8

The Director-General shall draw up a draft provisional agenda for each session of the Board, which shall be circulated to Member States and Associate Members within four weeks after the closure of its previous session.

Any proposal for the inclusion on the agenda of any item under (*c*), (*d*), and (*e*) of Rule 9 shall reach the Director-General not later than 10 weeks before the commencement of the session.

The provisional agenda of each session shall be drawn up by the Director-General in consultation with the Officers of the Board, on the basis of the draft provisional agenda and any proposals received under paragraph 2 of this Rule.

Where the Director-General and the Officers find it necessary to recommend the deferral or exclusion of proposals received under paragraph 2 of this Rule, the provisional agenda shall contain an explanation for such recommendation.

An annotated provisional agenda, together with any recommendations referred to in paragraph 4 of this Rule shall be dispatched with the notice of convocation to be sent in accordance with Rule 5 or Rule 6, as the case may be.

Rule 9

Except in the case of sessions convened under Rule 6, and subject to
Rule 8, the provisional agenda of each session shall include, inter alia:

(*a*) all items the inclusion of which has been ordered by the Health Assembly;

(*b*) all items the inclusion of which has been ordered by the Board at a previous session;

(*c*) any item proposed by a Member State or Associate Member of the
Organization;

(*d*) subject to such preliminary consultation as may be necessary between
the Director-General and the Secretary-General of the United Nations,
any item proposed by the United Nations;

(*e*) any item proposed by any specialized agency with which the Organization has entered into effective relations; and

(*f*) any item proposed by the Director-General.

Rule 10

Except in the case of special sessions convened under Rule 6, any
authority referred to in Rule 9 may propose one or more additional items of
an urgent nature for inclusion in a supplementary provisional agenda after
the deadline referred to in the second paragraph of Rule 8 and before the
opening day of the session. Any such proposal shall be accompanied by a
supporting statement from the authority initiating it. The Director-General
shall include any such item in a supplementary provisional agenda which
the Board shall examine together with the provisional agenda.

Rule 10 bis

The Board, subject to its constitutional mandate and having regard to the
resolutions and decisions of the Health Assembly, shall adopt its agenda at
the opening meeting of each session on the basis of the provisional agenda,
together with any supplement thereto. In adopting its agenda, the Board
may decide to add to, delete from, or amend, the provisional agenda and
any supplement thereto.

Rule 11

The Board shall not proceed, unless it determines otherwise, to the discussion of any item on the agenda until at least forty-eight hours have
elapsed after the relevant documents have been made available to the members.

OFFICERS OF THE BOARD

Rule 12

The Board shall elect its officers, viz. a Chairman, four Vice-Chairmen and one Rapporteur, from among its members each year at its first session after the Health Assembly, following a principle of rotation among geographical regions. These officers shall hold office until their successors are elected. The Chairman shall not become eligible for re-election until two years have elapsed since he ceased to hold office.

Rule 13

In addition to exercising such powers as are conferred upon him elsewhere by these Rules, the Chairman shall declare the opening and closing of each meeting of the Board, shall direct the discussions, accord the right to speak, put questions, announce decisions and ensure the application of these rules. The Chairman shall accord to speakers the right to speak in the order of their requests. He may call to order any speaker whose remarks are irrelevant to the subject under discussion.

Rule 14

If the Chairman is absent from a meeting or any part thereof, he shall designate one of the Vice-Chairmen to preside. The same procedure shall be followed when the Chairman is unable to attend a session of the Board.

If the Chairman is unable to make this designation, the Board shall elect one of the Vice-Chairmen to preside during the session or meeting.

Rule 15

If the Chairman for any reason is unable to complete his term of office, the Board shall elect a new Chairman for the remaining period of his term.

If the Chairman is unable to act in between sessions, one of the Vice-Chairmen shall act in his place. The order in which the Vice-Chairmen shall be requested to serve shall be determined by lot at the session at which the election takes place.

COMMITTEES OF THE BOARD

Rule 16

The Board may establish such committees as it may deem necessary for the study of, and reporting on, any item on its agenda. Standing committees established by the Board shall be composed of members of the Board or their alternates (referred to in these Rules as "committees of limited membership"). All Member States and Associate Members shall have the right to attend such committees in accordance with Rule 3. All committees other than standing committees shall be open-ended, composed of all interested Member States of the Organization (referred to in these Rules as "open-ended committees"), unless the Board decides otherwise, for a specific purpose and under exceptional circumstances.

The composition of committees of limited membership shall be determined by the Board, after hearing any proposals made by the Chairman, respecting the principles of equitable geographical representation, gender balance and balanced representation of developing and developed countries and countries in transition, having regard to the membership of the Board.

In committees of limited membership, the Chairmen and all other officers deemed necessary shall be determined by the Board or, in the absence thereof, by the committees themselves, respecting the principles of equitable geographical representation, gender balance and balanced representation of developing and developed countries and countries in transition. The Chairman and officers shall rotate regularly between regions and, wherever applicable, between developed and developing countries and countries in transition within the regions.

In open-ended committees, the Chairmen and any other officer deemed necessary shall be determined by the Board or, in the absence thereof, by the committees themselves, respecting the principles of equitable geographical representation, gender balance and balanced representation of developing and developed countries and countries in transition.

The Board shall review from time to time the need to maintain any committee established under its authority.

Rule 16 bis

Subject to any decision of the Board, and as provided in these Rules, the procedure governing the conduct of business and voting in committees established by the Board shall conform as far as practicable to the Rules relating to the conduct of business and voting in plenary meetings of the Board. Open-ended committees shall conduct their business on the basis of consensus. In the event of an inability to reach consensus, the difference of views shall be reported to the Board.

In the case of committees of limited membership, a majority of the members shall constitute a quorum.

No distinction in terms of rights of participation in open-ended committees shall be made between members of the Board and Member States not represented on the Board.

SECRETARIAT

Rule 17

The Director-General shall be *ex officio* Secretary of the Board and of any subdivision thereof. He may delegate these functions.

Rule 18

The Director-General shall report to the Board on the technical, administrative and financial implications, if any, of all agenda items submitted to the Board.

Rule 19

The Director-General or a member of the Secretariat designated by him may at any time make either oral or written statements concerning any question under consideration.

Rule 20

The Secretariat shall prepare summary records of the meetings. These summary records shall be prepared in the working languages and shall be distributed to the members as soon as possible after the close of the meetings to which they relate. Members shall inform the Secretariat in writing of any corrections they wish to have made, within such period of time as shall be indicated by the Director-General, having regard to the circumstances.

Rule 21

Reports of each session of the Board, containing all resolutions, recommendations and other formal decisions, as well as the summary records of the Board and of its committees, shall be communicated by the Director-General to all Member States and Associate Members of the Organization. Such reports shall also be submitted to the subsequent Health Assembly so that it may take such action as appropriate, for information, endorsement or approval, having regard to the respective functions of the Health Assembly and of the Board as set forth in the Constitution.

LANGUAGES [1]

Rule 22

Arabic, Chinese, English, French, Russian and Spanish shall be both the official and the working languages of the Board.

---

[1] See resolution WHA31.13.

Rule 23

Speeches made in an official language shall be interpreted into the other official languages in all meetings of the Board and of committees established by it.

Rule 24

Any member, or representative of a State Member or of an Associate Member, or of an invited non-Member State may speak in a language other than the official languages. In this case he shall himself provide for interpretation into one of the working languages. Interpretation into the other working languages by interpreters of the Secretariat may be based on the interpretation given in the first working language.

Rule 25

All resolutions, recommendations and other formal decisions of the Board shall be made available in the working languages.

CONDUCT OF BUSINESS

Rule 26

Two-thirds of the members of the Board shall constitute a quorum.

Rule 27

A member may at any time request his alternate designated in accordance with Article 24 of the Constitution to speak and vote on his behalf on any question. Moreover, upon the request of the member or his alternate, the Chairman may allow an adviser to speak on any particular point and, in the absence of the member or his alternate, if so requested in writing by the member or his alternate, to speak and vote on any question.

Rule 28

The Board may limit the time allowed to each speaker.

Rule 29

During the discussion of any matter, a member may rise to a point of order, and the point of order shall be immediately decided by the Chairman. A member may appeal against the ruling of the Chairman, in which case the appeal shall immediately be put to the vote. A member rising to a point of order may not speak on the substance of the matter under discussion but on the point of order only.

Rule 30

During the course of a debate the Chairman may announce the list of speakers and, with the consent of the Board, declare the list closed. He may, however, accord the right of reply to any member if in his opinion a speech delivered after he has declared the list closed makes it desirable.

Rule 31

The following motions shall have precedence in the following order over all other proposals or motions before the meeting, except a point of order:

(*a*) to suspend the meeting;

(*b*) to adjourn the meeting;

(*c*) to adjourn the debate on the item under discussion; and

(*d*) for the closure of the debate on the item under discussion.

Rule 32

Subject to Rule 31, any motion calling for a decision on the competence of the Board to adopt a proposal submitted to it shall be put to the vote before a vote is taken on the proposal in question.

Rule 33

During the discussion on any matter, a member may move the suspension or the adjournment of the meeting. Such motions shall not be debated, but shall immediately be put to a vote.

For the purpose of these Rules "suspension of the meeting" means the temporary cessation of the business of the meeting and "adjournment of the meeting" the termination of all business until another meeting is called.

Rule 34

During the discussion of any matter, a member may move the adjournment of the debate on the item under discussion. In addition to the proposer of the motion, one speaker may speak in favour of, and one against, the motion, after which the motion to adjourn the debate shall be immediately put to the vote.

Rule 35

A member may at any time move the closure of the debate on the item under discussion whether or not any other member has signified his wish to speak. If request is made for permission to speak against closure, it may be accorded to not more than two speakers, after which the motion shall be immediately put to the vote. If the Board decides in favour of closure the

Chairman shall declare the debate closed. The Board shall thereafter vote only on the one or more proposals moved before the closure.

Rule 36

A member may move that parts of a proposal or of an amendment shall be voted on separately. If objection is made to the motion for division, the motion for division shall be voted upon. Permission to speak on the motion for division shall be given only to two speakers in favour and two speakers against. If the motion for division is carried, those parts of the proposal or of the amendment which are separately approved shall subsequently be put to the vote as a whole. If all operative parts of the proposal or the amendment have been rejected, the proposal or the amendment shall be considered to have been rejected as a whole.

Rule 37

When an amendment to a proposal is moved, the amendment shall be voted on first. When two or more amendments are moved to a proposal, the Board shall first vote on the amendment deemed by the Chairman to be furthest removed in substance from the original proposal and then on the amendment next removed therefrom, and so on, until all the amendments have been put to the vote. Where, however, the adoption of one amendment necessarily implies the rejection of another amendment, the latter amendment shall not be put to the vote. If one or more amendments are adopted the amended proposal shall then be voted upon.

A motion is considered an amendment to a proposal, if it merely adds to, deletes from, or revises part of that proposal. A motion which constitutes a substitution for a proposal shall be considered as a proposal.

Rule 38

If two or more proposals are moved, the Board shall first vote on the proposal deemed by the Chairman to be furthest removed in substance from the proposal first presented and then on the proposal next removed therefrom, and so on, until all the proposals have been put to the vote, unless the result of a vote on a proposal makes unnecessary any other voting on the proposal or proposals still outstanding.

Rule 39

A motion may be withdrawn by its proposer at any time before voting on it has commenced, provided that the motion has not been amended or, if amended, that the proposer of the amendment agrees to the withdrawal. A motion thus withdrawn may be reintroduced by any member.

Rule 40

When a proposal has been adopted or rejected it may not be reconsidered at the same session unless the Board, by a two-thirds majority of the members present and voting, so decides. Permission to speak on a motion to reconsider shall be accorded only to two speakers opposing the motion, after which it shall be immediately put to the vote.

Rule 41

The Chairman may at any time require any proposal, motion, resolution, or amendment to be seconded.

VOTING

Rule 42

Each member of the Board shall have one vote. For the purpose of these Rules, the phrase "members present and voting" means members casting a valid affirmative or negative vote. Members abstaining from voting shall be considered as not voting.

Rule 43

Decisions by the Board on important questions shall be made by a two-thirds majority of the members present and voting. These questions shall include:

(a) recommendations on: (i) the adoption of conventions and agreements, (ii) the approval of agreements bringing the Organization into relation with the United Nations and intergovernmental organizations and agencies in accordance with Articles 69, 70 and 72 of the Constitution, (iii) amendments to the Constitution, (iv) the effective working budget, and (v) suspension of the voting privileges and services of a Member State under Article 7 of the Constitution; and

(b) decisions to suspend or amend these Rules of Procedure.

Except as otherwise provided by the Constitution of the Organization, or decided by the Health Assembly, or laid down in these Rules, the decisions of the Board on other questions, including the determination of additional questions to be decided by a two-thirds majority, shall be made by a majority of the members present and voting.

Rule 44

If the votes are equally divided on a matter other than an election the proposal shall be regarded as not adopted.

Rule 45

The Board shall normally vote by show of hands, except that any member may request a roll-call which shall then be taken in the alphabetical order of the names of the members. The name of the member to vote first shall be determined by lot.

Rule 46

The vote of each member participating in any roll-call shall be inserted in the records.

Rule 47

After the Chairman has announced the beginning of voting, no member shall interrupt the voting except on a point of order in connexion with the actual conduct of voting.

Rule 48

Elections shall normally be held by secret ballot. Except as concerns the nomination of the Director-General and the appointment of the Regional Directors, and in the absence of any objection the Board may decide to proceed without taking a ballot on an agreed candidate or list of candidates. Where a ballot is required, two tellers appointed by the Chairman from among the members present shall assist in the counting of votes.

The nomination of the Director-General shall be decided by secret ballot in accordance with Rule 52.

Subject to Article 54 of the Constitution, the appointment of a Regional Director shall be for five years and he or she shall be eligible for reappointment once only.

Rule 49

In addition to the cases provided for elsewhere by these Rules the Board may vote on any matter by secret ballot if it has previously so decided by a majority of the members present and voting, provided that no secret ballot may be taken on budgetary questions.

A decision under this rule by the Board whether or not to vote by secret ballot may only be taken by a show of hands; if the Board has decided to vote on a particular question by secret ballot, no other mode of voting may be requested or decided upon.

Rule 50

Subject to the provisions of Rule 52, when only one elective place is to be filled and no candidate obtains in the first ballot the majority required, a second ballot shall be taken which shall be restricted to the two candidates obtaining the largest number of votes; if in the second ballot the votes are equally divided, the Chairman shall decide between the candidates by drawing lots.

Rule 51

When two or more elective places are to be filled at one time under the same conditions, those candidates obtaining in the first ballot the majority required shall be elected. If the number of candidates obtaining such majority is less than the number of places to be filled, there shall be additional ballots to fill the remaining places, the ballots being restricted to the candidates obtaining the greatest number of votes in the previous ballot to a number not more than twice the places remaining to be filled.

Rule 52

At least six months before the date fixed for the opening of a session of the Board at which a Director-General is to be nominated, the Director-General shall inform Member States that they may propose persons for nomination by the Board for the post of Director-General.

Any Member State may propose for the post of Director-General one or more persons, submitting with the proposal the curriculum vitae or other supporting information for each person. Such proposals shall be sent under confidential sealed cover to the Chairman of the Executive Board, care of the World Health Organization in Geneva (Switzerland), so as to reach the headquarters of the Organization not less than two months before the date fixed for the opening of the session.

The Chairman of the Board shall open the proposals received sufficiently in advance of the session so as to ensure that all proposals, curricula vitae and supporting information are translated into all official languages, duplicated and dispatched to all Member States one month before the date fixed for the opening of the session.

If no proposals have been received by the deadline referred to in the second paragraph of this Rule, the Director-General shall immediately inform all Member States of this fact and that they may propose persons for nomination in accordance with this Rule, provided such proposals reach the Chairman of the Board at least two weeks prior to the date fixed for the opening of the session of the Board. The Chairman shall inform Member States of all such proposals as soon as possible.

All members of the Board shall have the opportunity to participate in an initial screening of all candidatures in order to eliminate those candidates not meeting the criteria proposed by the Board and approved by the Health Assembly.

The Board shall decide, by a mechanism to be determined by it, on a short list of candidates. This short list shall be drawn up at the commencement of its session, and the selected candidates shall be interviewed by the Board meeting as a whole as soon as possible thereafter.

The interviews should consist of a presentation by each selected candidate in addition to answers to questions from members of the Board. If necessary, the Board may extend the session in order to hold the interviews and make its selection. The Board shall fix a date for the meeting at which it shall elect a person by secret ballot from among the candidates on the short list.

For this purpose each member of the Board shall write on his ballot paper the name of a single candidate chosen from the short list. If no candidate obtains the majority required, the candidate who obtains the least number of votes shall be eliminated at each ballot. If the number of candidates is reduced to two and if there is a tie between these two candidates after three further ballots, the procedure shall be resumed on the basis of the short list originally established at the commencement of the balloting.

The name of the person so nominated shall be announced at a public meeting of the Board and submitted to the Health Assembly.

SUSPENSION AND AMENDMENT OF RULES OF PROCEDURE

Rule 53

Subject to the provisions of the Constitution and having regard to any relevant decisions of the Health Assembly, any of these Rules may be suspended by the Board in accordance with Rule 43, provided that at least forty-eight hours' notice of the proposal for such suspension has been given to the Chairman and communicated by him to the members twenty-four hours before the meeting at which the proposal is to be submitted. If, however, on the advice of the Chairman the Board is unanimously in favour of such a proposal, it may adopt it immediately and without notice. Any such suspension shall be limited to a specific purpose and to a period required to achieve that purpose.

Rule 54

Subject to the provisions of the Constitution, the Board may amend or supplement these Rules.

GENERAL PROVISIONS

Rule 55

The Board may at its discretion apply such Rules of Procedure of the Health Assembly as it may deem appropriate to particular circumstances for which provision does not exist in these Rules.

Appendices

Appendix 1

MEMBERS OF THE WORLD HEALTH ORGANIZATION
(at 31 December 2004)

The Members and Associate Members of the World Health Organization are listed below, with the date on which each became a party to the Constitution or the date of admission to associate membership.

Afghanistan	19 April 1948
Albania*	26 May 1947
Algeria*	8 November 1962
Andorra	15 January 1997
Angola	15 May 1976
Antigua and Barbuda*	12 March 1984
Argentina*	22 October 1948
Armenia	4 May 1992
Australia*	2 February 1948
Austria*	30 June 1947
Azerbaijan	2 October 1992
Bahamas*	1 April 1974
Bahrain*	2 November 1971
Bangladesh	19 May 1972
Barbados*	25 April 1967
Belarus*	7 April 1948
Belgium*	25 June 1948
Belize	23 August 1990
Benin	20 September 1960
Bhutan	8 March 1982
Bolivia	23 December 1949
Bosnia and Herzegovina*	10 September 1992
Botswana*	26 February 1975
Brazil*	2 June 1948
Brunei Darussalam	25 March 1985
Bulgaria*	9 June 1948
Burkina Faso*	4 October 1960
Burundi	22 October 1962
Cambodia*	17 May 1950
Cameroon*	6 May 1960
Canada	29 August 1946
Cape Verde	5 January 1976
Central African Republic*	20 September 1960
Chad	1 January 1961
Chile*	15 October 1948
China*	22 July 1946
Colombia	14 May 1959
Comoros	9 December 1975
Congo	26 October 1960

---

* Member States that have acceded to the Convention on the Privileges and Immunities of the Specialized Agencies and its Annex VII.

Cook Islands	9 May 1984
Costa Rica	17 March 1949
Côte d'Ivoire*	28 October 1960
Croatia*	11 June 1992
Cuba*	9 May 1950
Cyprus*	16 January 1961
Czech Republic*	22 January 1993
Democratic People's Republic of Korea	19 May 1973
Democratic Republic of the Congo*	24 February 1961
Denmark*	19 April 1948
Djibouti	10 March 1978
Dominica*	13 August 1981
Dominican Republic	21 June 1948
Ecuador*	1 March 1949
Egypt*	16 December 1947
El Salvador	22 June 1948
Equatorial Guinea	5 May 1980
Eritrea	24 July 1993
Estonia*	31 March 1993
Ethiopia	11 April 1947
Fiji*	1 January 1972
Finland*	7 October 1947
France*	16 June 1948
Gabon*	21 November 1960
Gambia*	26 April 1971
Georgia	26 May 1992
Germany*	29 May 1951
Ghana*	8 April 1957
Greece*	12 March 1948
Grenada	4 December 1974
Guatemala*	26 August 1949
Guinea*	19 May 1959
Guinea-Bissau	29 July 1974
Guyana*	27 September 1966
Haiti*	12 August 1947
Honduras	8 April 1949
Hungary*	17 June 1948
Iceland	17 June 1948
India*	12 January 1948
Indonesia*	23 May 1950
Iran (Islamic Republic of)*	23 November 1946
Iraq*	23 September 1947
Ireland*	20 October 1947
Israel	21 June 1949
Italy*	11 April 1947
Jamaica*	21 March 1963
Japan*	16 May 1951
Jordan*	7 April 1947
Kazakhstan	19 August 1992
Kenya*	27 January 1964
Kiribati	26 July 1984
Kuwait*	9 May 1960
Kyrgyzstan	29 April 1992

---

* Member States that have acceded to the Convention on the Privileges and Immunities of the Specialized Agencies and its Annex VII.

Lao People's Democratic Republic*	17 May 1950
Latvia	4 December 1991
Lebanon	19 January 1949
Lesotho*	7 July 1967
Liberia	14 March 1947
Libyan Arab Jamahiriya*	16 May 1952
Lithuania*	25 November 1991
Luxembourg*	3 June 1949
Madagascar*	16 January 1961
Malawi*	9 April 1965
Malaysia*	24 April 1958
Maldives*	5 November 1965
Mali*	17 October 1960
Malta*	1 February 1965
Marshall Islands	5 June 1991
Mauritania	7 March 1961
Mauritius*	9 December 1968
Mexico	7 April 1948
Micronesia (Federated States of)	14 August 1991
Monaco	8 July 1948
Mongolia*	18 April 1962
Morocco*	14 May 1956
Mozambique	11 September 1975
Myanmar	1 July 1948
Namibia	23 April 1990
Nauru	9 May 1994
Nepal*	2 September 1953
Netherlands*	25 April 1947
New Zealand*	10 December 1946
Nicaragua*	24 April 1950
Niger*	5 October 1960
Nigeria*	25 November 1960
Niue	4 May 1994
Norway*	18 August 1947
Oman	28 May 1971
Pakistan*	23 June 1948
Palau	9 March 1995
Panama	20 February 1951
Papua New Guinea	29 April 1976
Paraguay	4 January 1949
Peru	11 November 1949
Philippines*	9 July 1948
Poland*	6 May 1948
Portugal	13 February 1948
Qatar	11 May 1972
Republic of Korea*	17 August 1949
Republic of Moldova	4 May 1992
Romania*	8 June 1948
Russian Federation*	24 March 1948
Rwanda*	7 November 1962
Saint Kitts and Nevis	3 December 1984
Saint Lucia*	11 November 1980
Saint Vincent and the Grenadines	2 September 1983

* Member States that have acceded to the Convention on the Privileges and Immunities of the Specialized Agencies and its Annex VII.

Samoa	16 May 1962
San Marino	12 May 1980
Sao Tome and Principe	23 March 1976
Saudi Arabia	26 May 1947
Senegal*	31 October 1960
Serbia and Montenegro*	28 November 2000
Seychelles*	11 September 1979
Sierra Leone*	20 October 1961
Singapore*	25 February 1966
Slovakia*	4 February 1993
Slovenia*	7 May 1992
Solomon Islands	4 April 1983
Somalia	26 January 1961
South Africa*	7 August 1947
Spain*	28 May 1951
Sri Lanka	7 July 1948
Sudan	14 May 1956
Suriname	25 March 1976
Swaziland	16 April 1973
Sweden*	28 August 1947
Switzerland	26 March 1947
Syrian Arab Republic	18 December 1946
Tajikistan	4 May 1992
Thailand*	26 September 1947
The former Yugoslav Republic of Macedonia*	22 April 1993
Timor-Leste	27 September 2002
Togo*	13 May 1960
Tonga*	14 August 1975
Trinidad and Tobago*	3 January 1963
Tunisia*	14 May 1956
Turkey	2 January 1948
Turkmenistan	2 July 1992
Tuvalu	7 May 1993
Uganda*	7 March 1963
Ukraine*	3 April 1948
United Arab Emirates*	30 March 1972
United Kingdom of Great Britain and Northern Ireland*	22 July 1946
United Republic of Tanzania*	15 March 1962
United States of America	21 June 1948
Uruguay*	22 April 1949
Uzbekistan*	22 May 1992
Vanuatu	7 March 1983
Venezuela (Bolivarian Republic of)	7 July 1948
Viet Nam	17 May 1950
Yemen	20 November 1953
Zambia*	2 February 1965
Zimbabwe*	16 May 1980
Associate Members	
Puerto Rico	7 May 1992
Tokelau	8 May 1991

---

* Member States that have acceded to the Convention on the Privileges and Immunities of the Specialized Agencies and its Annex VII.

Appendix 2

STATUTE OF THE INTERNATIONAL AGENCY FOR RESEARCH ON CANCER[1]

Article I – Objective

The objective of the International Agency for Research on Cancer shall be to promote international collaboration in cancer research. The Agency shall serve as a means through which Participating States and the World Health Organization, in liaison with the International Union against Cancer and other interested international organizations, may cooperate in the stimulation and support of all phases of research related to the problem of cancer.

Article II – Functions

In order to achieve its objectives, the Agency shall have the following functions:

1. The Agency shall make provision for planning, promotion and developing research in all phases of the causation, treatment and prevention of cancer.

2. The Agency shall carry out a programme of permanent activities. These activities shall include:

   (*a*) the collection and dissemination of information on epidemiology of cancer, on cancer research and on the causation and prevention of cancer throughout the world;

   (*b*) the consideration of proposals and preparation of plans for projects in, or in support of, cancer research; such projects should be designed to make the best possible use of any scientific and financial resources and special opportunities for studies of the natural history of cancer which may arise;

   (*c*) the education and training of personnel for cancer research.

3. The Agency may arrange for the carrying out of special projects; however, such special projects shall be initiated only upon the specific approval of the Governing Council, based upon the recommendation of the Scientific Council.

---

[1] Approved by the Eighteenth World Health Assembly on 20 May 1965 (resolution WHA18.44). Pursuant to its Articles III and XI, the Statute entered into force on 15 September 1965. Amendments to the Statute adopted by the Governing Council at its seventh, ninth, twenty-seventh and thirty-first sessions in 1969, 1971, 1986 and 1990 respectively were accepted by the Twenty-third, Twenty-fifth, Thirty-ninth and Forty-third World Health Assemblies (resolutions WHA23.23, WHA25.25, WHA39.13 and WHA43.23).

4. Such special projects may include:

(*a*) activities complementary to the permanent programme;

(*b*) the demonstration of pilot cancer prevention activities;

(*c*) the encouragement of, and the giving of assistance to, research at the national level, if necessary by the direct establishment of research organizations.

5. In carrying out its programme of permanent services or any special projects the Agency may collaborate with any other entity.

Article III – Participating States

Any Member of the World Health Organization may, subject to the provisions of Article XII, participate actively in the Agency by undertaking, in a notification to the Director-General of the World Health Organization, to observe and apply the provisions of this Statute. In this Statute, Members which have made such a notification are termed "Participating States".

Article IV – Structure

The Agency shall comprise:

(*a*) the Governing Council;

(*b*) the Scientific Council;

(*c*) the Secretariat.

Article V – The Governing Council

1. The Governing Council shall be composed of one representative of each Participating State and the Director-General of the World Health Organization, who may be accompanied by alternates or advisers.

2. Each member of the Governing Council shall have one vote.

3. The Governing Council shall:

(*a*) adopt the budget;

(*b*) adopt financial regulations;

(*c*) control expenditure;

(*d*) decide on the size of the Secretariat;

(*e*) elect its officers;

(*f*) adopt its own rules of procedure.

4. The Governing Council, after considering the recommendations of the Scientific Council, shall:

(*a*) adopt the programme of permanent activities;

(*b*) approve any special project;

(*c*) decide upon any supplementary programme.

5. Decisions of the Governing Council under sub-paragraphs (*a*) and (*b*) of paragraph 3 of this Article shall be made by a two-thirds majority of its members who are representatives of Participating States.

6. Decisions of the Governing Council shall be taken by a simple majority of members present and voting, except as otherwise provided in this Statute. A majority of members shall constitute a quorum.

7. The Governing Council shall meet in ordinary session at least once in each year. It may also meet in extraordinary session at the request of one-third of its members.

8. The Governing Council may appoint sub-committees and working groups.

Article VI – The Scientific Council

1. The Scientific Council shall be composed of a maximum of twenty highly qualified scientists, selected on the basis of their technical competence in cancer research and allied fields.

2. The members of the Scientific Council shall be appointed by the Governing Council. The Director-General of the World Health Organization, after consultation with qualified scientific organizations, shall propose a list of experts to the Governing Council.

3. The members of the Scientific Council shall serve for a term of four years. However, the Governing Council may make appointments for a shorter term if this is necessary to maintain balanced annual rotation of members of the Scientific Council.

Any member leaving the Scientific Council, other than a member appointed for a reduced term, may be reappointed only after at least one year has elapsed.

Should any vacancies occur, a new appointment shall be made for the remainder of the term to which the member would have been entitled.

4. The Scientific Council shall be responsible for:

(*a*) adopting its own rules of procedure;

(*b*) the periodical evaluation of the activities of the Agency;

(*c*) recommending programmes of permanent activities and preparing special projects for submission to the Governing Council;

(*d*) the periodical evaluation of special projects sponsored by the Agency;

(*e*) reporting to the Governing Council, for consideration at the time that body considers the programme and budget, upon the matters dealt with in sub-paragraphs (*b*), (*c*) and (*d*) above.

Article VII – Secretariat

1. Subject to the general authority of the Director-General of the World Health Organization, the Secretariat shall be the administrative and technical organ of the Agency. It shall in addition carry out the decisions of the Governing Council and the Scientific Council.

2. The Secretariat shall consist of the Director of the Agency and such technical and administrative staff as may be required.

3. The Director of the Agency shall be selected by the Governing Council. The appointment shall be effected by the Director-General of the World Health Organization on such terms as the Governing Council may determine.

4. The staff of the Agency shall be appointed in a manner to be determined by agreement between the Director-General of the World Health Organization and the Director of the Agency.

5. The Director of the Agency shall be the chief executive officer of the Agency. He shall be responsible for:

(*a*) preparing the future programme and the budget estimates;

(*b*) supervising the execution of the programme and the scientific activities;

(*c*) directing administrative and financial matters.

6. The Director of the Agency shall submit a report on the progress of the Agency and the budget estimates for the next financial year to each Participating State and to the Director-General of the World Health Organization, which shall be distributed to reach them at least thirty days before the regular annual meeting of the Governing Council.

Article VIII – Finance

1. The administrative services and permanent activities of the Agency shall be financed by annual contributions by each Participating State.

2. These annual contributions shall be due on 1 January of each year and must be paid not later than 31 December of that year.

3. The level or levels of annual contributions shall be determined by the Governing Council.

4. Any decision to change the level or levels of annual contributions shall require a two-thirds majority of the Members of the Governing Council who are representatives of Participating States.

5. A Participating State which is in arrears in the payment of its annual contribution shall have no vote in the Governing Council if the amount of its arrears equals or exceeds the amount of contributions due from it for the preceding financial year.

6. The Governing Council may establish a working capital fund and decide its amount.

7. The Governing Council shall be empowered to accept grants or special contributions from any individual, body or government.

The special projects of the Agency shall be financed from such grants or special contributions.

8. The funds and assets of the Agency shall be treated as trust funds under Article VI (6.6 and 6.7) of the Financial Regulations of the World Health Organization.[1] They shall be accounted for separately from the funds and assets of the World Health Organization and administered in accordance with the financial regulations adopted by the Governing Council.

Article IX – Headquarters

The site of the headquarters of the Agency shall be determined by the Governing Council.

Article X – Amendments

Except as provided in Article VIII, 4, amendments to this Statute shall come into force when adopted by the Governing Council by a two-thirds majority of its members who are representatives of Participating States and accepted by the World Health Assembly.

Article XI – Entry into force

The provisions of this Statute shall enter into force when five of the States which took the initiative in proposing the International Agency for

---

[1] The relevant Article has been replaced by Regulation IX in the revised Financial Regulations (see page 93).

Research on Cancer have given the undertaking referred to in Article III to observe and apply the provisions of the present Statute.

Article XII – New Participating States

After the entry into force of this Statute, any State Member of the World Health Organization may be admitted as a Participating State, provided that:

(*a*) the Governing Council, by a two-thirds majority of its members who are representatives of Participating States, considers that the State is able to contribute effectively to the scientific and technical work of the Agency;

(*b*) and thereafter, the State gives the undertaking referred to in Article III.

Article XIII – Withdrawal from Participation

A Participating State may withdraw from participation in the operation of the Agency by notifying the Director-General of the World Health Organization of its intention to withdraw. Such a notification shall take effect six months after its receipt by the Director-General of the World Health Organization.

INDEX

INDEX

Accidental injuries, prevention, functions of, WHO, 2
Accidents to staff, compensation for, 102
Accounts of WHO, 10, 93, 94-95, 123, 143
Adjournment of debate, in Executive Board, 161
   in Health Assembly, 136, 137
Adjournment of meeting, in Executive Board, 161
   in Health Assembly, 136, 137
Adjournment of session of Health Assembly, 131
Administrative services, common, with United Nations, 46
   establishment and maintenance, functions of WHO, 2
Administrative Tribunal of the United Nations, 104
Advisers to Health Assembly delegates, 5, 126, 127
   to members of Board, 8, 37, 153, 160
Advisory committees on health research, 116, 120
Agenda, *see under* Executive Board, Expert Committees, World Health Assembly
Agreements, 2, 8, 48, 125
   adoption by Health Assembly, 7, 14, 16, 139
   annual reports by Member States on, 7, 15
   for agreements with individual organizations, see under name of organization
Aliens' registration, exemption, 27, 29
Allowances, expert committee members, 107
   staff, 45, 101, 102, 103
Alternates to Health Assembly delegates, 5, 126, 127
   to members of Board, 8, 37, 146, 153, 160
Amendments, to Constitution, 14, 16, 139, 149
   to proposals in Executive Board, 162, 163
      in Health Assembly, 134-135, 137, 138
   to rules of procedure, 149, 166
   to Statute of International Agency for Research on Cancer, 177
Americas, Region of the, 21, 38-40
Appeals by staff, 103-104
Appointment of staff, *see* Recruitment and appointment of staff
Appropriations, 88-89, 91, 96
Archives of specialized agencies, inviolability, 25
Arrest, immunity from, 27, 37
Assessments, 14, 89, 90-91, 144
   see also Contributions
Assistant Directors-General, appointment and salary, 101
   privileges and immunities, 37
Associate Members, admission, 20, 148
   contributions, 20, 144
   list, 172
   participation in Executive Board, 20, 153
      in Health Assembly, 4, 19, 123, 126, 127, 133